The Rhetorical Voice of Psychoanalysis

The Rhetorical Voice of Psychoanalysis

Displacement of Evidence by Theory

DONALD P. SPENCE

HARVARD UNIVERSITY PRESS
Cambridge, Massachusetts
London, England
1994

Library of Congress Cataloging-in-Publication Data
Spence, Donald P.
    The rhetorical voice of psychoanalysis : displacement of evidence
by theory / Donald P. Spence.
        p.   cm.
    Includes bibliographical references and index.
    ISBN 0-674-76874-4
    1. Psychoanalysis—Philosophy.   2. Psychoanalysis—Research.
3. Science—Methodology.   I. Title.
RC506.S663   1994
150.19′52′01—dc20   93-6344
                        CIP

To Edward Isham Spence McGregor

Acknowledgments

I am grateful for the encouragement of my friend and neighbor, Theodore Weiss, who read an early draft and clarified many matters of style and voice. Dr. Linwood Urban read the chapter on medieval and Aristotelian influences and made many useful suggestions. I am also indebted to my patients, whose refusal to accept empty or untimely interpretations sharpened my ear for the telling example and the appropriate moment. And I owe special thanks to Mrs. Ariel Moore, who brought the final manuscript into readable form with unfailing patience and dedication.

Contents

Introduction   1

I Background

   1. The Second Oedipal Tragedy   9
   2. Retreat from Galileo   27
   3. Aristotelian and Medieval Influences   48

II The Rhetorical Voice

   4. Metaphor as Theory   77
   5. Self-Analysis as Justification   97
   6. The Misleading Case Study   118

III Implications

   7. Happy Examples and Alternative Formulations 145
   8. Theories of the Mind: Fact or Fiction?   164
   9. A New Evidential Surface   183
   10. Two Kinds of Knowing   200

References   207
Index   217

We honor folk notions. But not because we believe in them. No, folk notions represent our collective, half-conscious effort to vivify the drab dailiness of our existence: they have a way of intensifying, of making more thrilling, whatever regularity we count on in order to plan our lives . . . The landscape of belief and that of fact are not opposed, or not diametrically, at least. No, they lie at some oblique angle to each other. Tired of the predictabilities that nourish, we long for that other world, the one we keep extrapolating, collectively, from scraps of belief. The landscape of belief relates to that of fact in rather the way the planet Pluto related, once, to Neptune. The orbit of the latter, or certain irregularities in it, let astronomers infer both the existence and location of a presence they'd never seen.

—Philip Garrison, *Augury*

Introduction

As psychoanalysis prepares to enter its second century, we are forced to realize that it is not much closer to being a science than it was when Freud first invented the discipline. Our accumulated clinical experience over the past one hundred years has given us no better demonstration of the central psychoanalytic assumptions than we find in Freud's original five cases. Clinical wisdom is largely stored as memory, we have not been able to assemble a public data base of clinical evidence, and a close look at crucial theoretical concepts makes it clear that they have little to do with clinical observations.

This troubling lack of progress can be laid to two factors: reliance on an outmoded method of scientific data collection and a preference for fanciful argument over hard fact. Writing to Jung in 1911, Freud admitted that he "was not at all cut out to be an inductive researcher— I was entirely meant for intuition." "Like a good rhetorician," writes one of Freud's critics, Freud "knew that the rhetorical counterpart of inductive proof in scientific demonstration was the example, whose logical frailty demanded the support and distraction of persuasive maneuvers." Freud began his scientific career in the orthodox manner by following traditional Baconian principles of inductive investigation, but at about the time he began to lose faith in his theory of seduction, he retreated to a more Aristotelian approach. He began to rely on choice specimens and favorite examples to make his point, he played down the importance of replication as a hedge against error, and he depended increasingly on arguments based on authority. Data remained secret and hidden from outside review and critique. In 1912

1

Freud announced that if the reader was not inclined to agree with his formulations, then additional data would scarcely change his mind. This position was a direct challenge to the core principles of the Baconian Revolution and the central importance of public participation in the process of science. In the years to follow, the form of psychoanalytic argument has tended to rely more on rhetorical persuasion than on appeal to data.

As the evidence became more anecdotal, rhetoric tends to make up for errors of measurement and observation. The rhetorical voice of psychoanalysis can be heard when Freud tells us that the central role of infantile wishes in dreams "cannot be contradicted as a general proposition"; that in his reconstruction of early experiences from the reports of his patients, he has "restored what is missing"; that "in mental life, nothing which has once formed can perish . . . everything is somehow preserved and . . . in suitable circumstances . . . can once more be brought to light." We hear the voice when Kurt Eissler tells us that Freud's self-analysis will "one day take a place of eminence in the history of ideas" and when Ernest Jones tells us that it was continued every day as long as Freud lived (one might ask, How can he be so sure?). We hear the voice when Charles Brenner writes that "like every other scientist, a psychoanalyst is an empiricist who imaginatively infers functional and causal relations among his data." And finally, we hear the rhetorical voice—somewhat ironically—when James Strachey tells us that Freud was "never rhetorical."

Sweeping statements of this kind are breathtaking in their persuasive appeal; we must fight hard not to be taken in by their rhetorical power. Once we look them straight in the eye, however, they begin to lose some of their force. But this is easier said than done, because Freud's choice metaphors are so appealing on literary grounds that it seems almost disrespectful to ask questions about the underlying evidence. And to ask such questions invites the loss of a much-beloved tradition.

When Freud abandoned his inductive training around the turn of the century and chose instead to present only illustrative examples to make his points, he left a mark on the form and content of clinical reporting that is still visible today. Followers of Freud seem to think that his anecdotal approach, with its focus on the convenient example, is the only way to do clinical science and that any attempt to follow traditional, Baconian procedures would violate a sacred trust. If we pick up any issue of a current psychoanalytic journal we find a friendly defense of standard theory, buttressed by one or more supporting anecdotes. Case reports are illustrative but always incomplete, and the level of argument is largely respectful and undemanding; logical errors are overlooked and there is no tradition of even-handed debate or continuing argument from one paper to the next.

Most disturbing of all is the absence of data. Anecdotal case reports highlight clinical observations that conform to expectation and tend to omit the unique or unexpected event. The complete clinical transcript is never presented; as a result, the reader can never draw his own conclusions from the evidence and must always give way to the views of the author. But this tradition seriously interferes with the possibility for friendly disagreement and tends to support the tradition of privileged withholding. Argument by authority stands directly in the way of the benefits, zealously guarded since the Renaissance, of an adversarial, critical, and dialectical tradition of investigation.

For an account of what may happen when scholars are denied open access to essential data, we need look no further than the history of alchemy during the Renaissance. It relied heavily on secrecy and magic and on restricted access to insiders or initiates, it communicated its findings largely in hermetic forms, and it discounted the importance of replication as an essential road to knowledge. This history shows us that once secrecy obtains a footing in the enterprise, it tends to elevate argument by authority and other rhetorical devices over the careful sifting of relevant evidence. As rhetoric displaces evidence, we lose the ability to reach what Jurgen Habermas has called an "uncompelled consensus." Protected by its use of secrecy, arcane language, and unprincipled rhetoric from the challenges of the disbeliever, alchemy and the occult in general became even more fallible and reached a dead end around the time of the Renaissance.

Is psychoanalysis headed in the same direction? Theory seems disturbingly disconnected from the data and unreasonably influenced by Freud. For evidence of this influence, we need look no further than the recent—and somewhat embarrassing—revision of the seduction theory. As is well known, Freud had originally believed reports by his female hysterical patients that they had been seduced by their fathers, but had revised his opinion around the turn of the century. In the new theory, he almost invariably described accounts of seduction as fantasies; psychoanalysts simply did not believe that such reports could be true. In the years from 1920 to 1976, not one paper appeared in the psychoanalytic literature with the word "seduction" in the title! Under the sway of Freud's authority, the profession was unable to evaluate the accumulating clinical evidence properly, and even went so far as to excommunicate one of its members who argued to the contrary, Jeffrey Masson. It is only in the very recent past that analysts have begun to realize that accounts of childhood seduction are not necessarily a product of the patient's imagination.

The seduction error is perhaps the most obvious example of the way in which theory can displace evidence. We can assume that fairly detailed clinical accounts of childhood seductions were available throughout the last one hundred years, but so strong was the official position (that seduction was a fantasy) that *no* paper was published up to 1976 that would argue to the contrary. We have, of course, no way of telling whether the fault lies with too-timid authors or too-cautious editors, but either way, it is disturbing to recognize the power of Freud's authority and the way in which theory prevails over observation. And the excommunication of Masson only continues the tradition begun by the expulsion of Jung, Adler, Horney, and Sullivan. Evidence that does not support standard theory tends to be minimized or disparaged, and independent thinking tends to be discredited.

Unless these traditions can be challenged and the power of rhetoric diminished, the fate of psychoanalysis as a creative enterprise would seem in jeopardy. Particularly disturbing is the fact that the seduction error was discovered from outside, not inside, the clinical hour (the shift in point of view was significantly influenced by the emerging feminist criticism of psychoanalysis). The failure of analysts to discover the error calls attention to the absence of self-correcting mechanisms in the application of the theory. The consequences of the mistake are equally disturbing. If a central doctrine, such as the role of fantasy in memories of seduction, can be so much mistaken, on what grounds can we continue to believe in such concepts as the unconscious, transference, and the Oedipus complex? If, as a recent survey has shown, there are relatively few good examples of clinically effective interpretations, there is reason to suspect the truth of other concepts as well. And if theory is largely unsupported by systematic clinical observations (as distinct from casually gathered anecdotal evidence), then we begin to see theory in a new light. Rather than representing an earnest and possibly fallible attempt to tell a true story about the world, psychoanalytic theory may function much more as a shared fantasy that binds its followers in a common belief system and protects them from uncertainty and doubt. As theory begins to merge with myth, we begin to understand why clinical evidence is only rarely reported and why challengers of received theory are treated as outcasts rather than as innovators.

The time has come to call attention to the rhetorical voice of psychoanalysis before it can do further damage and before more evidence is displaced by unsupported assumptions.

I

Background

1 The Second Oedipal Tragedy

Homeward bound on the high seas sometime during the last century, the man at the helm saw nothing wrong with believing that the earth was the center of the universe and was surrounded, like the skin of an orange, by a fixed shell of stars. He may have heard that this theory was wrong and that the earth was not, in fact, fixed but moving—at a speed of 18,000 miles a minute—through outer space. But he still found it both comforting and convenient to believe that Copernicus was wrong and Ptolemy was right: that the earth—and better yet, his ship—was at the absolute center of creation. Since the stars were fixed, he could take bearings from them at designated times and determine his position at the point where these bearings intersected. The sea might seem boundless and in continuous motion, completely devoid of fixed markers, but the sky, especially on a clear night, was filled with reliable guides.

Now that we know that the sun is the center of the solar system, we tend to see the Ptolemaic world view as a myth that has been corrected by science—an outdated belief system that has been replaced by a more satisfying theory. Yet the Ptolemaic world view is a useful myth for the navigator at sea because it excludes the complicating fact that the earth is always moving in space. By allowing him to pretend that the earth is still and surrounded by a blanket of stars, it simplifies his task of taking correct readings and fixing a position. In his comprehensive history of astronomy, Hogben writes that the Ptolemaic system "is still the most convenient representation of the apparent movements of the sun, moon, and fixed stars. It is the world view of the earth-observer, and as such remains the basis of elementary expositions on nautical astronomy after nearly two thousand years" (1943, p. 107).

At the same time, we also realize that belief in the Ptolemaic system would never allow us to send a probe to Jupiter, to understand red shifts from faraway stars, or to explore the beginning seconds of the universe. Its usefulness disappears as soon as we leave the atmosphere. To explore outer space, we need to know that the earth is moving along with the stars and planets and that when we look up at the sky on a dark night we cannot always trust our eyes.

Many aspects of psychoanalytic theory have something in common with the Ptolemaic world view. They provide us with short-term guidance in well-defined clinical situations, and because they often rest on simplifying assumptions, they enable us to concentrate better on the job at hand, but they are coming to be seen as inadequate for more far-reaching investigations. In a now-famous description, Freud referred to his theory of instincts as "our mythology . . . [a theory of] mythical entities magnificent in their indefiniteness. In our work we cannot for a moment disregard them, but we are never sure that we are seeing them clearly" (Freud, 1933, p. 95). To think of instincts as falling midway between the biological and the phenomenal is a useful myth because it puts certain kinds of clinical happenings into sharper focus, but we should never believe the myth in all its details.

It can be argued that the mythic aspects of psychoanalytic theory have both blinded us to its shortcomings and prevented it from operating, in true theoretical fashion, on a provisional and hypothetical basis. Because many of our theory/myths resonate with the central questions of man's place in the universe, we are persuaded by their narrative truth even as we disbelieve their details. The Oedipus myth, for example, owes much of its effectiveness to its ability to combine "the performative power of the clinical event and the performative power of the literary resonance" (Felman, 1983, p. 1048). It is a reasonably good description of a broad array of findings and thus clinically true and useful, but in addition, the myth brings with it distant echoes of the Sophocles text that are true in another sense—true of mankind. The strength of this second truth prevents us from treating the Freudian Oedipus story as just another hypothesis. From a nonexperimental point of view, it seems to tell us something important about the human condition.

The larger truth of the Oedipus story is both its strength and its weakness. To the extent that every male child, for reasons of biological necessity, *must* have both a father and a mother, the myth holds out the possibility that all men when they were young loved their mother and hated their father. This was Freud's original insight, expressed in an October 1897 letter to Fliess: "The Greek legend seizes upon a compulsion which everyone recognized because he senses its existence within himself. *Everyone* in the audience [of Grillparzer's play about incest and parricide] was once a budding Oedipus in fantasy and each recoils in horror from the dream fulfillment here translated into reality, with the full quantity of repression which separates his infantile state from his present one. Fleetingly the thought passed through my head that the same thing might be at the bottom of *Hamlet* as well" (Masson, 1985, p. 272; italics mine).

But the larger truth is also its weakness because it protects against the stray fact that threatens to negate it. The mythic side of the oedipal theory can too easily displace its more scientific side. And because the mythic side seems incontrovertible and universal, investigators tend to consider the matter closed and are less interested in uncovering a true accounting of how many male patients actually have sexual fantasies about their mothers, or in how many cases the successful completion of treatment depended on an analysis of such fantasies. It is partly for this reason that more systematic steps have not been taken to collect a usable data base and seek ways of confirming or disconfirming our central theories.

Because there is no public data base and no tradition of archival research, clinical findings have been stored primarily as memories in the minds of practicing analysts. In this somewhat porous state, they constitute a shifting and unreliable corpus that is permanently lost with the death of each practitioner. Even when the host is living, his memory is not exactly open to public inspection or consensual validation, nor is it available for the confirmation or disconfirmation of theoretical propositions. The details of these memories can never be checked against the facts, and we must assume that they are at the mercy of many of the distortions of remembering that Freud was the first to warn us against. How many of our good faith efforts to retrieve a clinical example in order to support this or that theoretical position are producing merely screen memories? In how many instances do we unwittingly fabricate a far-off clinical memory in our eagerness to support received theory? Because of its largely memorial nature, our accumulated clinical evidence is particularly vulnerable to the influence of largely unproven theory, and to an extent that can never be documented.

Because of our need to preserve the mythic nature of our more important theories and our failure to systematically accumulate a public data base (a failure supported by the need to protect our patients and ourselves from too-embarrassing questions), there has grown up, over time, a gradual decoupling of theory from evidence. Deprived of a common set of facts that might represent the gist of our collective wisdom, theory is free to tell whatever story it chooses. Deprived of the normal checks and balances of the average field of investigation, with its agreed-upon corpus of findings, psychoanalytic theory is free to fill the role of shared fantasy. Under the guise of theory, any number of scenarios can be imagined, published, and circulated, and the fate of these constructions will depend more on the Zeitgeist and on the personal history of the theorist than on the data (because the data are largely out of sight).

For an example of how theory can be projected (and protected) in a way that is uncluttered by actual facts, we might consider the following well-known description of the "good hour" in psychoanalysis:

> Let me start with a schematic example. It concerns an experience which, though not frequent, is familiar to all analysts. And it is one welcome to all. I mean "the good analytic hour." Its course is varied, and I offer only an abstraction from experiences well advanced in analytic therapy. Many a time the "good hour" does not start propitiously. It may come gradually into its own, say after the first ten or fifteen minutes, when some recent experience has been recounted, which may or may not refer to yesterday's session. Then a dream may come, and associations, and all begins to make sense.
>
> In particularly fortunate instances a memory from the near or distant past, or suddenly one from the dark days may present itself with varying degrees of affective charge. At times new elements are introduced as if they had always been familiar, so well do they fit into the scheme of things. And when the analyst interprets, sometimes all he needs to say can be put into a question. The patient may well do the summing up by himself, and himself arrive at conclusions. (Kris, 1956, pp. 446–447)

This is an engaging narrative that manages, in the absence of a single clinical observation, to convince us of the possibility of the "good hour" and acquaint us with the conditions under which it comes into existence. Kris has created a specimen out of words alone; it is neither fact nor fiction but has some of the attributes of both. He presents us with a fantasy we would all like to share but describes it in a way that makes it sound real. But a close inspection of his account shows us that the details will always remain just out of sight. The memory from the "near or distant past" is left vague and undescribed, the "affective charge" is left unstated, and the way in which all the pieces fit into the "scheme of things" is left to our imagination. Even the final interpretation—perhaps only a question—goes unstated, along with the final summing up by the patient.

The description casts a mythic spell because it is presented in the form of a coherent narrative with the classic marks of an uneasy beginning (it "does not start propitiously") and a happy ending ("the patient may well do the summing up by himself"). It tells a tale we would all like to share; as a result, we tend to read it in a largely uncritical manner. In the short space of a well-constructed paragraph, the "good hour" has come into being, and so artful is the presentation that many readers remember the passage as being about an actual clinical occurrence. But persuasion, it should be noted, is brought about by means of the rhetorical voice, not the evidential voice.

Something else happens as well—something even more disabling. As each reader ponders the earmarks of the good hour, he or she will very likely imagine moments in his or her own clinical experience that came close to fitting Kris's description. The fact that these moments are stored as memories allows them to be more easily fitted into the master scheme than if they were hard data, and it can be imagined that an attempt to reach agreement on a "good hour" from a series of verbatim possibilities would very likely end in failure. When familiar with Kris's account, the reader may very likely decide that it matches his or her experience. In this manner, the classic account of the "good hour" has been vindicated by each new reader, and its state changed from provisional/hypothetical to one of consensual validation. But this seeming achievement is only a trick of memory and language; we are still at the mercy of the rhetorical voice.

For a controlled demonstration of how popular theory can influence memory, we can go back to a landmark experiment by Lillian Robbins, which concerned the way in which early child-rearing practices are misremembered by parents only a few years after the fact (Robbins, 1963). Retrospective reports of standard child-rearing events were compared with clinic records, and significant distortions were found in the recall of such items as when the infant stopped using the bottle, when bowel training was begun, when bladder training was begun, and when the 2 A.M. feeding was stopped. The errors, particularly those made by the mothers, tended to follow the advice of Dr. Benjamin Spock as presented in his best-selling book on child rearing, *Baby and Child Care* (1945). The parallel between the expert's advice and the prevailing direction of distortion strongly suggests that the mothers' memories were influenced by a highly visible theory.

Memories of Early Sexual Abuse

Not only can theory influence memory and bring about the same distortion in the clinician's account as Freud discovered in his patients' memories, but it can also cause other data, not consistent with the theory, to be significantly overlooked. In the very act of listening to a clinical hour in order to make it conform to received theory, we can easily fail to register one or more alternative meanings. Something like this seems to have happened to Freud at the start of his career as he listened to his patients' accounts of childhood sexual abuse. The advent of the oedipal theory seems to have triggered a sudden disappearance of these accounts, and the erosion can be systematically documented by a careful study of the Freud-Fliess letters (see Masson, 1985) and a review of the psychoanalytic literature from 1920 to the present. We start with the Fliess letters.

As is well known, it was a set of eighteen cases that first alerted Freud to the strong likelihood that "premature sexual experience" was the cause of hysteria. In a paper delivered to the Society of Psychiatry and Neurology in Vienna in April 1896, he announced that he had discovered an aetiological precondition for hysterical symptoms. The cases could be divided into three groups: 1) assaults and abuse at an early age, mostly practiced on female children; 2) longer-lasting adult-child love-relationships; and 3) sexual relations between children of opposite sexes. These eighteen cases formed the main thrust of his presentation to the Society and confirmed Breuer's original hypothesis that "the symptoms of hysteria are determined by certain experiences of the patient's which have operated in a traumatic fashion" (Freud, 1896, pp. 192–193). It could now be stated (with no if's, and's or but's) that "at the bottom of every case of hysteria there are *one or more occurrences of premature sexual experience,* occurrences which belong to the earliest years of childhood but which can be reproduced through the work of psychoanalysis in spite of the intervening decades" (Freud, 1896, p. 203; author's italics in the original).

As Schimek (1987) has recently pointed out, the set of eighteen original cases is only sketchily described in Freud's original paper, and as a result, we have no way of knowing exactly what he was told. We are limited to one long paragraph (1896, pp. 207–208), and even though Freud tells us that the findings are in a position to "speak for themselves," close inspection of the details reveals no specific information. The reader is thus in no position to draw his or her own conclusions. This is our first inkling of a less-than-adequate public data base, and we will find this state of affairs repeated many times throughout the history of psychoanalysis. Theory, it would seem, comes first, evidence a distant second. And even when theory changes in a drastic manner, as we will see shortly, the evidence is almost never called into question.

The reaction of the Society to Freud's excited discovery was cool at best. There seems to have been no discussion of the paper (see Masson, 1984, p. 6) and in a letter to Fliess in April 1896, shortly after the meeting took place, Freud describes his reception as "icy." He mentions only one detail — a "strange evaluation by Krafft-Ebing: 'It sounds like a scientific fairy tale.' And this, after one has demonstrated to them the solution of a more-than-thousand-year-old problem, a *caput Nili*. They can go to hell, euphemistically expressed" (Masson, 1985, p. 184).

Despite the cool, perhaps even chilly reception, Freud maintained a continuing interest in the hypothesis that childhood sexual experiences were a precondition for hysteria, and he continued to send examples to Fliess. In the forty-three letters written between the time of the Society meeting and his famous confession that he no longer believed in his "neurotica" (September 21, 1897), we can find eleven that either allude to the hypothesis or contain additional evidence in its support. Many years later, Freud tells us that his theory "broke down under its own improbability, and under contradiction in definitely ascertainable circumstances" (1914, p. 17), but this description hardly applies to the excitement of 1896 and 1897. On the contrary, he was collecting new examples almost until the time he went on his vacation in August of 1897, and we might wonder whether his subsequent recollection can be seen as another example of the "Robbins effect"—another instance of the way in which memory can be eroded in the service of theory.

If the theory did indeed collapse under its own improbability, the break was a long time coming. Allusions to or instantiations of the theory occurred in two letters in December 1896, and four in January, one in February, one in April, two in May, and one in June 1897. Freud must still have continued to believe that the hypothesis was important and salvageable and that new evidence was worth collecting and reporting to Fliess. These letters by themselves strongly suggest that Freud was not devastated by the cool reception he received from the Society.

But after Freud's confession that he no longer believed in his patients' reports (September 21, 1897), the flow of new examples almost completely stopped. In the forty-three letters that follow his confession (to match the forty-three from before), there is only one new example of an early memory of sexual abuse. In this letter (December 22, 1897), Freud describes a patient who has early memories of her parents' sexual activity from age seven months to sixteen years. In this, perhaps his most detailed clinical example, Freud gives us a graphic picture of a psychotic father who brutally cohabited with his wife, infected her with gonorrhea, and probably attempted anal intercourse despite her shouts, curses, and tears. And all in front of the daughter.

In the letters to follow, there are occasional references to Freud's "dreckology reports," but these seem largely related to his self-analysis and may have become the raw material for *Die Traumdeutung,* on which he was currently working. For whatever reason, they were usually referred to rather than directly quoted. There are no further supporting examples from his patients, but it was not until 1905 that Freud conceded in public (as opposed to his private speculation to Fliess) that actual seductions are no longer required to "arouse a child's sexual life." But he attenuates the force of his September 21 confession in the following cautious account: "I cannot admit that in my paper on the 'Aetiology of Hysteria' I exaggerated the frequency or importance of that influence, though I did not know that persons who remain normal may have had the same experience in their childhood, and though I consequently overrated the importance of seduction in comparison with the factors of sexual constitution and development" (1905, pp. 190–191).

Can we conclude, with Masson (1984, p. xxi), that Freud's "abandonment of the seduction hypothesis [was] a failure of courage"? This conclusion (which, when first announced, accounted in part for Masson's removal as director of the Freud Archives in 1981) does not do justice to either the complexity of the theoretical climate or to Freud's change of heart. In the first place, as Schimek (1987) and others have made clear, Freud never completely abandoned his seduction theory; as he states in his 1905 paper, he may have "overrated" the importance of early sexual experiences but he remained convinced of their functional significance. And the long delay between his September 21, 1897, confessional letter and his public statement would suggest that the change in approach was the result of a combination of factors and not simply a "failure of courage." At least two other considerations need to be brought into the picture.

In the first place, the role of the oedipal theory needs extended discussion, and from a point of view somewhat different from what is customary. In the usual account, the abandonment of the seduction hypothesis opened the way to the discovery of the Oedipus complex and Freud's realization of the all-important role of psychic reality as a critical theoretical concept. In the minds of some, if Freud had continued to believe in the seduction theory, he could never have created psychoanalysis. In her letter to Masson on September 10, 1981, Anna Freud tells him that "keeping up the seduction theory would mean to abandon the Oedipus complex, and with it the whole importance of fantasy life, conscious or unconscious fantasy. In fact, I think there would have been no psychoanalysis afterwards" (Masson, 1984, p. 113). But a close reading of the Freud-Fliess letters suggests that it was the other way around: that the oedipal theory, in part because of its mythic fascination and in part because it provided a more satisfactory all-around explanation, as we will see, may have tempted Freud to hear the clinical evidence in a slightly different manner, and that this response, in turn, brought about a different attitude toward its publication.

We have already pointed to the fact that the sample of forty-three letters, written to Fliess after he admitted that "I no longer believe in my *neurotica*," contains only one new instantiation of the seduction theory. If we assume that the diagnostic composition of his case load would not have changed in any significant manner in the months following the September letter to Fliess compared to the months before, we can then conclude that early memories from his patients, which seemed to support the seduction theory, would have continued at about the same pace. But if this were true, why should the rate of early sexual "sightings" drop from 23 percent (ten positive letters out of forty-three) to 2 percent? Assuming that the clinical information remained more or less constant, how can we explain the change in Freud's reporting style?

Personal Equation

It is time to turn to the importance of the personal equation in theory formation. Is there any evidence that the sudden shift from seduction theory to oedipal theory in 1897 was brought about for partly (or even entirely) autobiographical reasons? Our suspicions that this might be the case are raised by the sudden nature of the change and its timing, by the fit between the oedipal hypothesis and Freud's family of origin, and by the fact that neither of Freud's most sympathetic biographers is able to provide a convincing explanation.

Before turning to the commentaries, let us first consider the time-table. The date of his famous confession to Fliess about no longer being a believer is September 21, 1897; Freud's father died on October 23, 1896, the previous fall. On either the night *before* or the night *after* the funeral (see Freud 1900, p. 318, fn. 1), Freud dreamed about a printed notice or poster that contained the following messages:

"You are requested to close the eyes."
"You are requested to close an eye."

His associations led to the thought of overlooking or "winking at" an oversight—ostensibly, the somewhat unorthodox details of the rather plain funeral. But could the oversight also be a reference to the seduction theory? If it was universally found that all fathers routinely seduce their children, Jakob must have committed the act with his daughters, before Freud was born. It might have seemed necessary—particularly on the heels of his death—to overlook his father's likely involvement with his children and so let him rest in peace. At the time of his death, the oedipal theory was not yet in place, but if some way could be found to spare the father, Freud's task of mourning would be made that much easier.

But the alternative was not obvious, and early into the next year, Freud still seemed convinced that the father was to blame. In a letter to Fliess on February 11, he writes that "unfortunately my own father was one of these perverts and is responsible for the hysteria of my brother and those of several younger sisters. The frequency of this circumstance makes me wonder" (Masson, 1985, pp. 230–231). In hindsight, we can sense in the last sentence the beginning of the turn toward the idea that fantasy lies at the root of these reports because if they are found everywhere, they must be imaginary. But the final formulation still eluded him.

On May 31 of the following year, Freud tells Fliess that he had been dreaming of his oldest daughter Mathilde (age nine) and feeling "over-affectionate feelings" toward her: "The dream of course shows the fulfillment of my wish to catch a *Pater* as the originator of neurosis and thus puts an end to my ever-recurring doubts" (Masson, 1985, p. 249). In other words, the seduction theory still holds sway.

We next come to the famous letter of September 21 to Fliess in which Freud announces that "I no longer believe in my *neurotica*." What is perhaps most impressive about this date is that it was the day after Freud returned from his summer vacation (see Jones, 1953, p. 325). He had been away from patients for most of August and September; therefore, it was probably not a change in the clinical material that led to his reformulation. More than likely, it grew out of the fruits of his self-analysis and, as also seems likely, his continued doubts about his father (Jones draws the same conclusion; see p. 325). The Mathilde dream added his own guilt to the equation. If childhood seduction by the father was (as he had assumed) a universal failing, then he and his father were both guilty.

His earlier conviction that his patients had been seduced may have been stimulated in part by a need to punish his father, but in the wake of his father's death, and on the heels of evidence that he, Freud, may also have been guilty of the same crime, it seemed all the more necessary to find some alternative explanation. One escape from this dilemma was to blame himself, which he does in the letter of October 3. He writes to Fliess that "the old man plays no active part in my case, but that no doubt I drew an inference by analogy from myself onto him" (Masson, 1985, p. 268). Freud seems to be saying (perhaps with the Mathilde dream in mind) that he is the guilty party and that these feelings were projected onto his father, who should remain blameless.

By October 15 he goes a step further and makes the "universal" crime entirely imaginary. In a letter to Fliess on that date, he writes that "a single idea of general value dawned on me. I have found, in my own case too, [the phenomenon of] being in love with my mother and jealous of my father, and I now consider it a universal event in early childhood . . . If this is so, we can understand the gripping power of *Oedipus Rex*" (Masson, 1985, p. 272).

At this point in the story, it may be useful to consider some auto-biographical details. As is well known, Freud was the son of a young mother (twenty-one) and a father twenty years older. It is therefore tempting to argue that the circumstances of his early life might well have sensitized him to the possibility of oedipal rivalry.

We will never know, of course, exactly what train of circumstances led to the oedipal reformulation, but it seems clear that it was moti-vated in no small measure by personal reasons—not solely, as Freud indicates in his letter to Fliess, because of clinical concerns. Once the oedipal theory was firmly in place, Freud's doubts about his father and himself could be laid to rest. Our suspicion that personal reasons provide the primary pretext for the new theory is borne out not only by these facts, but by his assumption that he had discovered a universal law and by his continued refusal to consider any alternative.

> As he grew older, Freud hardened his views and increasingly saw the Oedipus complex as the center post of the entire structure of psy-choanalysis. When it came to discussion, his attitude was distinctly subjective. Thus when the Vienna Psychoanalytic Society discussed the infantile Oedipus complex years later, Freud opened the pro-ceedings 'by remarking that the point is to *demonstrate* the presence in the child of the Oedipus complex'—not, as might have been expected of a self-styled scientific body, to consider whether or not it was present . . . Even the least critical observer might wonder why the task was not to investigate rather than to establish. (Clark, 1980, p. 170)

Freud's two most sympathetic biographers write a somewhat dif-ferent story. Referring to the letter of September 21, Jones simply states that now "Freud had discovered the truth of the matter . . . This other side of the picture [that children had incest wishes toward the parent of the opposite sex] had been quite concealed from him. The first two months of his self-analysis had disclosed it" (1953, p. 322). In speaking of the "truth of the matter" that was "disclosed" by his self-analysis, Jones makes it seem as if the oedipal theory was a true discovery and says nothing about the possibility that it was a kind of compromise formation, a way of integrating the fruits of his dreams and fantasies with his clinical findings to reach a solution that maximized credibility and minimized discomfort.

James Strachey takes a similar position in his introduction to *Die Traumdeutung,* written in 1953. He tells us that "the existence of the Oedipus complex was only established during the summer and autumn of 1897" (Freud, 1900, pp. xviii–xix). Use of words like *existence* and *established* make it sound as if a real discovery had been accomplished. The casual reader would never know from this introduction that the nature of the theory is still widely contested and, in some quarters, simply not accepted.

Peter Gay, for his part, focuses his attention on clinical and theoretical issues (see Gay, 1988, p. 94). In his letter to Fliess of September 21, 1897, Freud makes four observations. First, he claims that he was either losing patients or only partially succeeding in his treatment. Second, the seduction theory, if universal, must therefore implicate all fathers and this seemed unlikely (and would necessarily raise questions about his own). Third, since the unconscious cannot distinguish between fact and fantasy, it is not necessarily triggered by an actual event. And fourth, not all the contents of the unconscious necessarily become conscious. Gay prefers to place the blame on the clinical material rather than on Freud's more personal concerns. As Toews (1991) makes clear, he "does not want to portray Freud as driven in his 'scientific' endeavors by the need to assuage his psychic suffering, to find meaning for his agonizing personal dilemmas, and to create a story that would make sense of his experience" (pp. 516–517). But as we have seen, the latter reading would seem to do the most justice to the material—both from his personal life and from his practice—and be most in keeping with the essential spirit of psychoanalysis.

We now get a further understanding of the relation between the early clinical evidence, the sudden shift away from the seduction theory, and the virtual blackout on contrary evidence up until the 1970s. If the oedipal theory is indeed a universal law, then it brooks no exceptions and stands with the discoveries of Galileo and Darwin among the foremost discoveries of mankind. Freud the discoverer becomes a hero who was able to recover from scientific failure with the greatest amount of glory. To maintain this piece of narrative truth, Freud and his followers are forced to emphasize the universal nature of the complex and maintain a skeptical attitude toward any negative evidence (see Clark, 1980, for further examples of this tendency). They were, in addition, in no position to find any evidence for the now-disowned seduction theory, since this would only raise questions about the need to abandon it with such haste.

But the oedipal complex is not a universal law, as Fisher and Greenberg (1977) make clear. In their review of the experimental studies up to 1977, they find that studies of young children *do not* support the shift in attitude toward opposite-sex parents the oedipal theory would predict (p. 182). Young children of *both* sexes tend to feel closer to their mother than their father. At some later point, each sex tends to identify more with the same-sex than with the opposite-sex parent, but the resolution of the oedipal complex seems to occur more out of identification than fear. Parts of the oedipal theory are thus upheld, but there is no data showing that, even in its qualified form, it can be considered a universal law.

Additional exceptions to the standard formulation have been noted by Emde (1992). Citing extensive supporting documentation, he lists the following limitations:

1. The superego is not an outcome of the resolved Oedipus complex and there is considerable moral development before the age of three.
2. Gender identity is not an outcome of the Oedipus complex.
3. Female development "is not secondary or less powerful than male development during the age period of the Oedipus complex. Freud was a product of his time and culture and focused on male development as prototypic with female development somehow secondary and more complex" (p. 352).
4. Variations in the family environment play a major role in the unfolding of the Oedipus complex.
5. The standard portrayal of the child's experience is oversimplified. Instead of appearing later on the scene, fathers seem to develop "early and qualitatively separate affectionate relationships with both young boys and girls" (p. 353).

In a recent review of the evidence, Bennett Simon tells us that "the research has in general made things more complicated, more intricate, and so far less amenable to relatively simple psychoanalytic theorizing" (1991, p. 662). But what is even more to the point, very little of this research has found its way into the mainstream journals. In the eyes of the official psychoanalytic establishment, the Oedipus complex today is little different from what it was a hundred years ago. Its unchanging nature again reminds us more of myth than of science, a reading supported by the fact that there is no good agreement on an exact definition or on how one would go about collecting relevant data (see Simon, 1991, p. 663).

As far back as 1915, one of Freud's critics observed that "the real sin which [he] has committed is: that when he found a certain phenomenon occurred sometimes, he said it occurred always. What we want to know is the proportion of times in which it occurs" (Ross, in a letter to *British Medical Journal;* cited in Clark, 1980, p. 172). We still have no good data on what proportion of patients seem to fit the standard oedipal classification or on how necessary the resolution of the standard oedipal complex is for a successful course of treatment.

What Kind of Science?

The history of this piece of theory clearly shows the drawbacks of the prescientific, Aristotelian position that has become all too characteristic of psychoanalysis. What began as an attempt to reconcile clinical findings with personal beliefs and combine them into a kind of theoretical compromise formation has endured—pretty much unchanged—up to the present time. What was (possibly) true for one man has become elevated to a general law. Few attempts have been made to discover the truth of this generality because such an effort, if conscientiously carried out, would necessarily point to flaws in Freud's own research and might raise questions about his need to maintain the status quo for a mixture of personal and professional reasons. While it may be unfair to describe these nonefforts as a kind of organized cover-up, there is no doubt that the psychoanalytic establishment seems less than enthusiastic about presenting an evenhanded account of the events that led to the replacement of the seduction theory by the oedipal theory, or make any attempt to discover the generality of the law, the extent to which the so-called "oedipal period" is a predictable developmental phase, or the extent to which the resolution of the Oedipus complex is a necessary precondition for successful treatment.

The full implications of the oedipal position staked out by Freud are still making themselves felt. By resorting to argument by authority to make his case, by claiming that the Oedipus complex was universal and thereby discouraging any systematic attempts to look at the evidence, Freud sent the message that data are ephemeral and not to be taken seriously, that they should be sacrificed to the privacy of the patient. It is probably no accident that the eighteen cases he assembled to support his seduction theory are the last example of Freud operating as a standard model, Royal Society scientist. He never again attempted to reason in strict inductive fashion from a series of cases; from that time on, he seemed more comfortable within a largely single-case, intuitive tradition. Evidence was clearly secondary, and in one of his early papers he argued that if the reader was not inclined to agree with his formulations, then additional data would scarcely change his mind (Freud, 1912, p. 114).

If evidence was secondary, theory was king, and as we have seen, it quickly became decoupled from the evidence. It is well known that one piece of the evidence—the clinical data on incest—is only just now being allowed to be recognized in its own right, to the continuing shame of the psychoanalytic establishment. A close look at the history of this error has recently been provided by Simon (1992), who makes clear how easy it is to use theory as a way of screening out facts and random observation as a means of supporting theory. It is well known among philosophers of science that, given world enough and time, the zealous investigator can *always* find confirmation for *any* theory.

If theory is not systematically grounded in the bedrock of observation, it can quickly turn into myth, and self-promoting and self-protecting myth at that. As myth replaces real knowledge, we have the beginning of a scientific tragedy—the tragedy in the title of this chapter—one set in motion by Freud when he opted for an explanation that was based on personal need and private circumstance, an explanation that was not supported by the data at large and not open to public question and debate.

By opting for a "universal" oedipal theory in place of the clinical evidence supporting seduction, Freud turned his back on the central assumptions of Royal Society science and effectively moved psychoanalysis out of the twentieth century into a period much closer to the Renaissance, which is where we are today.

After nearly a hundred years of experience with the analytic method, we still know surprisingly little about features of its natural landscape. Here is another way in which theory gets in the way of knowledge: because we think we know, we do not take the trouble to really look. We know next to nothing about how the analytic process unfolds, the impact of interpretations on psychic structures (to what degree and within what time frames), how to identify key features of the analytic surface to which the analyst seems to respond, how mutative interpretations differ from inexact mistakes, how critical memories change over time, and a host of similar, very specific, and largely unstudied issues. We are desperately in need of the equivalent of a Hubble telescope to investigate the analytic space and the analytic surface and to pick up important features of interest that undoubtedly keep recurring across sessions and across treatments.

But research of any significance in psychoanalysis today is like Mark Twain's weather—everyone talks about it but. . . . It would seem that much of the reluctance to look closely at the evidence in our field is not caused by our primarily clinical orientation, by the lack of trained investigators, or by the lack of funds. The reluctance also stems from a fear of being disloyal to Freud and even to our authoritarian tradition. To discover that the Oedipus complex is not what it seems is to make more than a scientific statement—it is also to condemn Freud for his early compromise. Somehow it is felt that in acting as less than a pure scientist, he was morally defective, and that loyal followers should never look in this direction again. But so long as the past is sealed over, I think it will continue to haunt us, and the way the psychoanalytic establishment tends to downplay research is one nontrivial consequence.

Not long after the publication of Freud's *Interpretation of Dreams*, another pioneer, Abraham Flexner, was writing a landmark critique of American and Canadian medical education, and his advice, despite its age, has a significant bearing on our present predicament.

> Medicine is a discipline in which the effort is made to use knowledge procured in various ways in order to effect certain practical ends. With abstract general principles [read metapsychology] it has nothing to do. It harbors no preconceptions as to diseases or their cure. Instead of starting with a finished and supposedly adequate dogma or principle, it has progressively become less cocksure and more modest. It distrusts general propositions, a priori explanations, grandiose and comforting generalizations. It needs theories only as convenient summaries in which a number of ascertained facts may be used tentatively to define a course of action. It makes no effort to

use its discoveries to substantiate a principle formulated before the facts were even suspected [worth underlining]. For it has learned from a previous history of human thought that men possessed of vague preconceived ideas are strongly disposed to force facts to fit, defend, or explain them. And this tendency both interferes with the free search for truth and limits the good which can be extracted from such truth. (1910, p. 156)

2 Retreat from Galileo

Writing to Fliess while putting the final touches on *Die Traumdeutung,* Freud compared his view of the book to a walk in the country. "At the beginning, the dark forest of authors (who do not see the trees), hopelessly lost on the wrong tracks. Then a concealed pass through which I lead the reader—my specimen dream with its peculiarities, details, indiscretions, bad jokes—and then suddenly the high ground and the view and the question: which way do you wish to go now?" (Masson, 1985, p. 365).

Freud begins the fifth chapter with a related metaphor. "Having followed one path to its end, we may now retrace our steps and choose another starting-point for our rambles through the problems of dream-life" (1900, p. 163). He returns to the same image in the final chapter, "The Psychology of the Dream Process," when he looks back at what has been done so far: "For it must be clearly understood that the easy and agreeable part of our journey lies behind us. Hitherto, unless I am greatly mistaken, all the paths along which we have travelled have led us towards the light—towards elucidation and fuller understanding. But as soon as we endeavor to penetrate more deeply into the mental process involved in dreaming, every path will end in darkness" (p. 511; see Mahony, 1987, for further discussion of these passages).

The expedition into the unknown—a popular genre for nineteenth-century travel writers and explorers—has become, in Freud's hands, a central image for the investigation of dreams. He is on his way to becoming our explorer of the mind, and his imaginary journey into this make-believe realm becomes a new kind of natural history. Two worlds are being explored at the same time, the literature of dreams

27

and what they are supposed to mean in the preliminary chapters of *Die Traumdeutung;* and the world of his unconscious as uncovered through his groundbreaking self-analysis, which was taking place around the time he was writing the book. Access to one world—his inner world—provides the maps and guidebooks that allow him to explore the other. Freud is our guide to the dark continent of the mind and we impatiently wait for each new report from the field.

As Freud joins the ranks of the other nineteenth-century explorers and travel writers, he takes us out of the neurology clinic and the physiology laboratory and into the unknown. The explorer's virtues—courage, perseverance, tolerance for discomfort—become his and endow his reports with a special urgency and passion for the truth. He has returned safely with a bag of specimens from the dark continent. Study his exhibits carefully because they have never been seen before. Heed well what he has to say because he is the first—and perhaps the last and only—witness.

Here is a parallel report from another explorer of about the same period:

> The next day I attempted to penetrate some way into the country . . .
> Finding it nearly hopeless to push my way through the wood, I fol-
> lowed the course of a mountain torrent. At first, from the waterfalls
> and number of dead trees, I could hardly crawl along: but the bed
> of the stream soon became a little more open, from the floods having
> swept the sides . . . The gloomy depth of the ravine well accorded
> with the universal signs of violence . . . I followed the watercourse
> till I came to a spot where a great slip had cleared a straight space
> down the mountain side. By this road I ascended to a considerable
> elevation and obtained a good view of the surrounding woods.
> (Darwin, 1890, pp. 220–221)

The similarity between the two accounts may not be entirely coincidental, because Darwin was one of Freud's heroes. In his autobiography, Freud wrote that "the theories of Darwin, which were then of topical interest, strongly attracted me, for they held out hopes of an extraordinary advance in our understanding of the world" (1925, p. 8).

By casting his study of dreams in the form of an exotic walk in an unexplored forest, Freud establishes himself as the naturalist and explorer who will discover the way into the mind itself and uncover its secrets. He invites the reader to follow but not necessarily either to verify or to replicate; we can go along on the journey but he remains the leader and guide. *Die Traumdeutung* is closer in form to Conrad's *Heart of Darkness* than to Robert Boyle's *Sceptical Chymist*. The tradition of participatory science, begun by Bacon and the Royal Society, is set to one side in favor of the elite explorer and the one-of-a-kind expedition. The reader is told (and shown) what was found, with the strong implication that this path will never be traveled again. Future explorers may make their way to the dark continent, but they will probably never again land at quite the same place.

Freud by this time was no stranger to the laboratory; thus it is more than a little surprising that in midcareer, he would all but abandon his roles as bench experimenter and clinical investigator to join the ranks of the descriptive scientists. As a young student working in a comparative anatomy lab, Freud's first project was to uncover the gonadic structure of the eel. He dissected some four hundred eels in the course of this work, and although he could not arrive at any definite conclusion and in the end felt dissatisfied with the research, the number of specimens alone is impressive. During the six years he spent at Brücke's laboratory, Freud gained experience in routine investigation with current techniques and developed new procedures of his own (such as a new staining procedure using gold chloride). Among his projects were the study of spinal cord cells in a certain species of fish and an analysis of the nucleus of the acoustic nerve.

Even after he left the laboratory and turned to more clinical research, Freud was still working very much in the classical Baconian, inductive tradition. In 1891 he published a study of thirty-five cases of hemiplegia in cerebral palsy. The next year one of his students carried out a study of fifty-three cases of diplegic forms of cerebral palsy for his dissertation. In this tradition, certainty was vested in repeated observation; any experimenter worth his salt was dedicated to the law of large numbers and the belief that a single observation was worthless but an accumulation of observations marked the road to the truth.

Freud was fond of claiming that his work as a traditional scientist, focused on traditional topics, received nothing but praise, in contrast to his later work, which was more often criticized. But in fact, as Henri Ellenberger points out, his work on cerebral palsy was criticized as well as praised. "An anonymous book review argued that Freud had described the pathological anatomy of [cerebral diplegia] not from his own observations but from a compilation of the findings of other authors which made Freud's physiopathological interpretations unconvincing, because the connection suggested by Freud between certain groups of symptoms and certain etiological factors were not sufficiently substantiated by the facts" (1970, p. 477; I am also indebted to Ellenberger for my summary of Freud's more traditional scientific career).

It is against this background of painstaking laboratory and clinical research, sometimes criticized for being too speculative, that Freud developed rather different methods when he turned to the study of the mind. A variety of reasons to account for this change have been uncovered, and I will discuss them later in the chapter. But whatever the final explanation may be, it seems clear that his role as explorer and naturalist protected him from certain kinds of criticism and allowed him to present only as much evidence as he thought appropriate. Although dream *specimens* were collected and described, they did not have quite the same properties as slides or sections; even though the dreams were converted into prose, the dream as dreamt (and its visual aspects in particular) was still not available for public inspection. Thus, Freud's conclusions could never be directly challenged because no one else could ever have the same dream or arrive at the same set of associations. A traveler in a foreign landscape that could never be visited twice in the same place, Freud was in a position to command respect for his observations but never have them questioned.

This overly protective attitude toward data has characterized psychoanalysis ever since. Evidence in psychoanalysis has always been difficult to verify. There is no archive of verbatim case reports to which we can turn; only a small number of analyzed cases (five) were published by Freud, and extended samples of verbatim analyst-patient dialogue are conspicuous by their absence. Freud's self-analysis has never been published, and we actually hear more about it from his biographers (who use it as a springboard for any number of undocumented conjectures) than from Freud himself. Taken as a whole, the psychoanalytic literature tends to minimize evidence at the expense of conclusion and maximize argument at the expense of evidence, and these tendencies can be laid directly at Freud's door.

But if the reader could not see for himself, his natural skepticism was largely overcome by Freud's flair for detail. What he discovered was so clearly presented in *Die Traumdeutung* that its reality became a foregone conclusion. In the new natural history of the mind, vision is still the primary sense and the discoveries along the way become as clear and as immediate as the findings of any other explorer. Even the relatively abstract seventh chapter of *Die Traumdeutung* is vivid with concrete detail and striking metaphor, and makes use of such analogies as comparing the process of condensation to printing a text in spaced or heavy type (p. 595), or comparing the systems of the mind to the lenses of a telescope (p. 611). Seeing becomes understanding; as each piece of the dark continent is brought into the light of day, ambiguity is dispelled and certainty takes over.

So vivid is Freud's language, and so commanding his presence as explorer and discoverer, that it is hard to realize that much of what he is describing cannot be seen at all. The history is "natural" in name only. The stuff of the mind is not there to be seen, and thus corroboration is out of the question. But swayed by the richness of the highly visual language and by the conviction expressed in its presentation, we soon forget that Freud is only outlining a hypothesis about the workings of the mind. In his role as guide and adventurer, he seems no different from other world explorers: what he tells us must, therefore, be true.

Clifford Geertz has written at length about the way an ethnographer can oscillate between the two roles of biographer and scientist. His task "demands both the Olympianism of the unauthorial physicist and the sovereign consciousness of the hyperauthorial novelist, while in fact not permitting either" (1988, p. 10). Geertz sees not only the conflict between the two roles but also the way in which one complements the other. The strong sense of "being there" that is brought about by the accumulation of incident tends to lend credence to what is observed. We see this happen as we read the opening lines of *We, the Tikopia* by Raymond Firth, a classic piece of anthropology from the 1930s:

> In the cool of the early morning, just before sunrise, the bow of the *Southern Cross* headed towards the eastern horizon, on which a tiny dark blue outline was faintly visible. Slowly it grew into a rugged mountain mass, standing up sheer from the ocean; then as we approached within a few miles it revealed around its base a narrow ring of low, flat land, thick with vegetation. The sullen grey day with its lowering clouds strengthened my grim impression of a solitary peak, wild and stormy, upthrust in a waste of waters.

In an hour or so we were close inshore and could see canoes coming round from the south, outside the reef, on which the tide was low. The outrigger-fitted craft drew near, the men in them bare to the waist, girdled with bark-cloth, large fans stuck in the backs of their belts, tortoise-shell rings or rolls of leaf in the ear-lobes and nose, bearded, and with long hair flowing loosely over their shoulders. Some plied the rough heavy paddles, some had finely plaited pandanus-leaf mats resting on the thwarts beside them, some had large clubs or spears in their hands. The ship anchored on a short cable in the open bay off the coral reef. Almost before the chain was down the natives began to scramble aboard, coming over the side by any means that offered, shouting fiercely to each other and to us in a tongue of which not a word was understood by the Mota-speaking folk of the mission vessel. I wondered how such turbulent material could ever be induced to submit to scientific study. (Firth, 1936, pp. 1–2; quoted in Geertz, 1988, p. 13)

Geertz summarizes this classic account of the natives of Tikopia in the following overview: "All the fine detail, marshaled with Dickensian exuberance and Conradian fatality—the blue mass [of the Polynesian island], lowering clouds, excited jabberings, velvet skins, shelved beach, needle carpet, enstooled chief—conduce to a conviction that what follows, five hundred pages of resolutely objectified description of social customs . . . can be taken as fact" (p. 13).

The same argument can be made about Freud on his imaginary journey. Even though the visual detail is a trick of language, it still operates to convince us of the truth of what we are reading. Even though his expedition explores the soft stuff of dreams, his presence as guide and leader becomes so persuasive that hypothesis quickly turns into certainty. In the years to come, he would forsake the role of explorer for that of archeologist, adding even greater realism to his findings; the Viennese naturalist now becomes a new kind of scientist and the stuff of the mind becomes the findings from an excavation. This role, which remained with him throughout his life, still lies ahead. For the moment, he is still an explorer of what lies on the surface, on the lookout for the high ground from which every prospect pleases.

What brought about the identification with explorer in the first place? At least two kinds of influence seem important. Almost every biographer has identified Freud's fascination with Hannibal, the conqueror of Italy, and there is evidence that this preoccupation dates back to his adolescence. In choosing Hannibal as his mentor, "Freud found an outlet for his political passions which served him well both emotionally and intellectually ... His own Oedipal rivalry had assumed a political form in his Hannibal fantasy, and so he adopted an openly counterpolitical stance aimed at freeing himself from the power politics exercised on his inner feelings" (McGrath, 1986, pp. 22–23). But Hannibal was not only a political power, he was also an explorer and adventurer, and while McGrath (and other biographers) emphasize the former aspect of Freud's identification, we should not forget Hannibal's many achievements as leader and trailblazer, the discoverer of new roads to Rome across the Alps.

The second kind of influence comes from more immediate surroundings. During the time he was writing *Die Traumdeutung*, Freud was spending long summers in the mountains making regular (and strenuous) ascents. He climbed Rax Alpe, a six-thousand-foot peak, three times in some weeks and noted his times up (three and a half hours) and down (two and a half hours) (see Clark, 1980, p. 198). Nearing the end of *Die Traumdeutung* in August of 1899, Freud wrote to Fliess to say that he was coming into the home stretch. "Things are incomparably beautiful here; we take walks, long and short, and all of us are very well, except for my occasional symptoms. I am working on the completion of the dream book in a large, quiet, ground-floor room with a view of the mountains There are some mushrooms here as well, though not yet many. The children naturally join in the hunt for them" (Masson, 1985, p. 363). Since he was exploring the woods, fields, and mountains when he could, it is not surprising that he used the same imagery to investigate the world of dreams and the dimly seen unconscious. Freud was confessedly "a connoisseur of scenery with an eye for the niceties of a great view, and embedded deep within his psyche there was a compelling need for intimate contact with nature" (Clark, 1980, p. 197).

Before leaving these examples of detailed description, it may be useful to call attention to their formal name, because it will play a significant part in later chapters. In choosing to frame significant sections of *Die Traumdeutung* in vivid pictorial language, Freud was making use of the classical figure of *enargia* and falling back on a long-standing rhetorical recommendation. Persuasion, it was thought, depended critically on bringing the target scene *ante oculos,* into the mind's eye. The "highest of all oratorical gifts," wrote one authority, consists in crafting the vivid illustration that "thrusts itself upon our notice," making the listener feel that "the facts on which he has to give his decision are . . . displayed in their living truth to the eyes of the mind" (Quintilian; cited in Vickers, 1988, p. 322; see also Mahony, 1987, for further discussion of this particular figure of speech). We will encounter enargia many more times in the pages to come; we mark it here because it signals our first encounter with the more literary aspect of the rhetorical voice of psychoanalysis.

An Intellectual Adventure Story

A careful reading of *Die Traumdeutung* not only reveals a passion for detail and its visual aspect, it also impresses us with an interpretative certainty that adds significantly to our feeling that Freud is on the scene and bringing back a first-person report. Interpretations are not cast as hypotheses but as definite conclusions. "Let me now," he writes, "put the dream thoughts in place of the dream" (p. 416). "Analysis made it possible to find another solution" (p. 457). "It is unnecessary, I think, to accumulate further examples [we might think back to the sample of almost four hundred eels!]. They would merely serve to confirm what we have gathered from those I have already quoted—that an act of judgment in a dream is only a repetition of some prototype in the dream-thoughts" (p. 459). These statements are not conditional or approximate or probabilistic; they are stated as definite findings, as if to say: these are the facts. Again and again, argument is grounded in certainty. Item: "We can have no hesitation in deciding in favor of the second alternative. There can be no doubt that the censoring agency . . . is also responsible for interpolations and additions [to the dream]" (p. 489). Item: "We must conclude that during the night the resistance loses some of its power . . ." (p. 526). Item: "I have now completed the interpretation of the [specimen] dream" (p. 118). To put the matter in these terms is to make interpretation as definitive and clearly structured as a walking tour of the Schladminger Tauern.

One source of this interpretative certainty seems to be the repeated use of the rhetorical figure enargia, which implements Freud's decision to cast *Die Traumdeutung* as a "ramble" through an unknown forest and heightens the realism of his walking imagery. These images, sometimes explicit, more often just below the surface, help to provide the concrete background for the objective field trip, thus adding significantly to the reader's sense of being there and being shown. Seeing himself as explorer and guide may also have helped Freud set aside the doubts he was expressing to Fliess. There is a striking change in tone between the letters to Fliess—written while he was drafting the dream book—and the final version of *Die Traumdeutung*. In his letters he was frequently unsure, perplexed, or close to despair. From March 10, 1898: "It was no small feat on your part to see the dream book lying finished before you. It has come to a halt again, and meanwhile the problem has deepened and widened. It seems to me that the theory of wish fulfillment has brought only the psychological solution and not the biological—or, rather, metapsychical—one" (Masson, 1985, p. 301). From May 1, 1898: "I have now written the section on psychology in which I had gotten stuck, but I do not like it, nor will it remain. The chapter you have now is stylistically still quite crude and bad in some parts, that is, written without much liveliness" (Masson, 1985, p. 312). But once the undertaking had been set in type, doubts were replaced by conviction. Anxious, uneasy speculation changed to quiet certainty.

The overlay of conviction helps to disguise the fact that Freud is thinking much of the time in quite a revolutionary manner. The rules of the primary process are not described until we reach the seventh chapter, a summary of the psychology of the dream process, but long before we get there we are presented with examples of primary-process thinking. In the more-extended examples (such as his analysis of the Botanical Monograph dream), we are treated to a dazzling parade of images that are semantically and experientially linked. The linkages are not entirely lawful, but the idiosyncrasy of both the examples and his interpretation of them is forgotten in the sheer drama of the display. And it is probably no accident that the journey through the botanical monograph, with its folded color plates and wide range of specimens, can be seen as a variation on a walk with a naturalist through an exotic jungle. Freud is still our guide, and through his eyes we see that people (Gartner, Flora) can be plants, that memories of a monograph on Cyclamen can be an allusion to Freud's love of books, and, most important of all, that the word *bookworm* can be read in at least two ways: as insect and as man (that is, the young Freud).

We have reached a new kind of high ground. In moving from fact to metaphor and by invoking the domain of language *(la langue)* as an organizing principle, Freud has moved beyond the simple appearance of things. Behind the thing lies the word, and the word can remind us of another word or perhaps, another meaning. We are no longer moving horizontally across the forest floor; Freud has shown the way to vertical links as well. From the pine forest of the Austrian Alps, we are transported to a tropical rain forest that surrounds us with associations, both semantic and phonetic, and opens our eyes to linkages we have never seen before. Vision is still the dominant medium and we are seeing everything for the first time. We begin to accept the fact that to go from Cyclamen to coca plant to Koller to glaucoma to Konigstein (as he does in his analysis of the Botanical Monograph dream, p. 171) is no more unlikely than to go from dried specimen to herbarium to bookworms to artichokes. And while the primary process may not seem entirely logical (and, as we learn later, cannot be), it soon feels familiar and believable.

We are also impressed by Freud's success in finding the answer. Each dream that comes his way is taken apart, scrutinized, rearranged, and reduced to a set of simpler propositions. *Die Traumdeutung* can be seen as a special kind of expedition—a sort of intellectual *Pilgrim's Progress* in which each obstacle to understanding is systematically overcome. We begin to admire Freud's ability to find a solution to each new puzzle; no detail seems too bizarre to defeat explanation. As an intellectual adventure, *Die Traumdeutung* is second to none, and as each obstacle is overturned, we cannot help but relax our critical evaluation of its scientific merits and find ourselves carried along by the exotic details of each new dream.

Credibility is also enhanced by the use of the word *specimen*. By presenting the dreams in italics and referring to them by a botanical term, Freud is suggesting that the dream text is just as distinct an object of study as a dried leaf or a petrified tree and implying that the dream as reported is somehow equivalent to the dream as dreamt. (In actuality, of course, we have no assurance that the text being studied is in any way isomorphic with the dream as dreamt).

Freud's associations are equally problematic. They are presented as if they stem naturally from the dream text, but we would suspect that they are equally influenced by the particular time and place of the dream analysis, and we have no information about these particulars. Thus we have no assurance that the associations could be replicated on some other occasion or that the source of a particularly inspired association might depend more on the context of a particular time and place than on the details of the dream.

If we read *Die Traumdeutung* as an intellectual exploration and adventure story, we lose sight of the fact that the *principle* of dream analysis keeps changing from one dream to the next and that, although each obstacle is overcome as soon as it appears, we do not systematically accumulate wisdom about how the overall task should be carried out. If we step back from some of the more bravura performances—the analysis of the specimen Irma dream, the two readings of the Botanical Monograph dream, the Count Thun dream, and one or two others—we see that these are one-of-a-kind expeditions that cannot be repeated. No one, it seems clear, when presented with any one of these dreams, would ever discover exactly the same paths through the network of associations. In the first place, the associations belong largely to Freud and thus are not available to any outside reader; in the second place, the methods used cannot be reduced to a set of rules. Although the seventh chapter was an attempt to set out the most important of these rules—the mechanisms of the primary process—it quickly becomes clear that the principles described there do not exhaust the intricacies of dream analysis and that no matter how carefully they are followed by another analyst, the process would not result in another *Traumdeutung*. Traveling in Freud's expedition does not make us better explorers; we only become more impressed by his resourcefulness and determination, and through a kind of rhetorical slight of hand, we conclude that skill in mastering the dream particulars must somehow produce knowledge of more general principles. But this list is always just out of reach. Failure to map the rules of performance onto the performance itself is an old story in the history of the humanities, and most critics have become accustomed to the slippage that exists between, say, Aristotle's laws of tragedy and the way these laws are carried out in *Hamlet* or *The Death of a Salesman*. But *Die Traumdeutung* is presented to us as science, not art, and the examples of dream interpretation as final accounts of dream meanings. *Deutung* means both interpretation and explanation, and the dominant tone of the book, as we have seen, supports the second usage. But careful consideration makes it clear that these readings cannot be definitive. In the first place, they reach no natural stopping point, which argues for the fact that the shorter examples might have been extended and that any one of the attempts might have been repeated at *another* time, perhaps reaching somewhat different conclusions (as was the case, in fact, with the two readings of the Botanical Monograph dream). Second, as I have already noted, the network of associations presented seems very much a function of the time and place of the interpretation; in other words, each reading may be a victim of its immediate context. Third, the fact that elements of the dream can be shown to form a network does not necessarily mean that it was this network that caused the dream; Freud may be confusing associations caused *by* the dream with the causes *of* the dream. And finally, the interpretations, no matter how dazzling, do not fulfill the role of an ideal explanation: they do not provide an account for each and every dream element, nor do they reduce the total fabric of the dream to a deep structure and a set of transforming operations.

For all of these reasons, the dreams so richly illustrated and analyzed in *Die Traumdeutung* serve mainly to illustrate how dream analysis *might* be carried out. They cannot stand as definitive explanations of a lawful and logical process. Yet this failure is lost sight of in the excitement of following Freud on the journey through each network of associations. In our haste to keep up with the leader, we may lose sight of the fact that his choice of path is often arbitrary and almost never discussed. Such deliberations would become a luxury in the fury of the chase, jeopardizing both the success of the expedition and our faith in the leader. Doubts might be expressed to Fliess but not to the public at large, and certainly not to his followers.

It is important to note that we are not being misled. It was the habit of the great explorers to keep some secrets to themselves, and while they clearly intended to amuse, entertain, and enlighten the reader, they did not promise to equip him to carry out his own expedition. We read Richard Burton or Charles Darwin with admiration for their exploits and fascination for their faraway ports of call but not with an eye to learning from their example. We may even find such details as equipment lists or techniques for staining specimens somewhat out of place; they bring us with a kind of rude awakening into a reality we would rather not enter. They do not fit into the hypnotic vision created by the author, just as a view of HMS *Beagle*, once we see how small it was, tends to diminish the sweep of Darwin's adventure.

Return to Aristotle

In exchanging the role of laboratory neurologist who dissected the gonads of some four hundred eels for the role of naturalist explorer who returned from a newly discovered country with a bag of exotic specimens, Freud was moving from one kind of science into another. Forsaking the new empiricism that had been gaining ground since the Renaissance, he was retreating to the more Aristotelian approach that was in danger of being displaced. Where the new science saw truth as resulting from a series of observations, no one of them critical, the old science saw nature to be transparent and truth self-evident. As Ramzy (1956) noted, "Aristotle believed that things appear to us as they are, that the human mind is constructed in such a way as to supply us with a valid picture of the external world. Truth is not outside the universe, it is under our eyes. The first instance of science is experience; it is the observation and study of natural phenomena" (p. 120). Ramzy was one of the first commentators to recognize the non-Galilean side of Freud's scientific outlook, but he also noted that this influence was, up to that time, "unduly neglected and even intentionally underestimated" (p. 118). The same point can be made at the present time, more than thirty years later. The formulations of both Adolf Grünbaum (1984) and Peter Gay (1988) encourage a view of Freud as a classical Galilean scientist and all but ignore the Aristotelian influence on his work. Their treatment of Freud's scientific outlook agrees almost perfectly with the strongly positivistic reading of Jones (1953), despite the recovery, during the intervening years, of many documents that tell quite a different story. I will come back to the reasons for this positivistic emphasis in a later chapter.

By bringing the study of dreams under the shelter of the old science, Freud was able to highlight the single specimen and play down the law of large numbers. The more Aristotelian approach allowed him to dwell on the particularities of the specific dream and its surrounding associations. Knowledge was contained in the details, and Aristotle (and more specifically his later followers) taught their students to believe that more could be learned from the study of a single specimen than by the accumulation of dozens of observations. This model suited the role of the naturalist explorer who was not equipped to carry out a controlled experiment but who had the job of reporting faithfully about everything that came his way.

Patrick Mahony (1987) has made a similar observation about Freud's scientific style: "Whereas he admittedly lacked talent for the inductivism of empirical psychology . . . he had intuitive powers and knew how to join his courage to their service. He coupled his admiration for those 'who have the courage to think something before they can demonstrate it' and his awareness of universal implications in the singular fact. He himself tells us how he saw a general relevance and applicability in the isolated case of Anna O." (pp. 167–168). Writing to Jung in 1911, Freud admits that "I was not at all cut out to be an inductive researcher—I was entirely meant for intuition" (cited in Mahony, p. 17). While we may suspect that part of the emphasis in this confession was designed to appeal to Jung's more mystical side, we cannot entirely discount its autobiographical truth.

In asking what kind of a scientist Freud thought himself to be and in trying to place him within a larger historical perspective, it may be useful to compare the two views of science that had been prevalent since the Renaissance. The first, or *conceptualist* view, originated with Aristotle and took nature to be essentially transparent and therefore completely intelligible. "Direct access to the essence or structure of natural objects is available, by a careful analysis of everyday concepts such as *motion* or *continuum,* for example, or through an insight on the part of a skilled investigator into the singular objects of sense, an insight sufficiently penetrating to allow the universal to be immediately grasped in them" (McMullin, 1967, p. 333). According to this view, surface revealed everything and was not distinguished from interior. "For Aristotle the immediate perceptible appearance, that which present-day biology terms the *phenotype,* was hardly distinguished from the properties that determine the object's dynamic relations" (Lewin, 1931, p. 149).

Worth noting is the fact that some investigators are more skilled than others; thus it follows that failure to appreciate the importance of new discoveries does not cast doubt on the validity of the discovery, as would be the case in the sciences of today, but is only a sign that the discoverer has powers or insights that place him apart from the ordinary experimenter. There is an elitism implicit in this view of science that can also be found in contemporary psychoanalysis. It is this elitism that allows the widespread use of argument by authority, because if we assume that only certain observers will be able to penetrate the transparency of the natural world, then there is every reason to listen to their verdict.

Once a correct discovery is made—and once it is properly phrased—then its claim to truth will be self-evident: "If it is properly understood—and getting to understand it may be no simple affair—the connection between its concepts will be seen to be of a necessary sort. The warrant is intrinsic in the statement; once the latter is properly understood, there will be no need to look outside it for further evidence" (McMullin, 1967, p. 333). This doctrine can be seen to argue against the need to collect further observations; at the same time, it justifies the most painstaking study and restudy of approved discoveries because only in this way can we extract their full measure of wisdom. Favorite specimens are collected and passed down from one generation to the next because they are seen to represent the discovery in a way that is particularly apt or telling. They are cherished, furthermore, because they cannot be replaced by more abstract principles.

By contrast, the newer *empiricist* view of science took the position that the natural world was too opaque to be directly penetrated by human insight. If transparency could not be assumed, then knowledge would come about only as a result of careful and persistent observation, and any particular result would only approximate the final solution. Evidence was derived from an accumulation of observations; it was not found in concepts or examples. Preliminary findings might be cast in the form of hypotheses, but these were convenient fictions that, sooner or later, would be superseded by further observations. And no matter how intriguing they seemed, these hypotheses could never be evaluated by careful study or commentary; no mere inspection of a statement could decide its truth value. As a result, the empiricists saw no reason to collect specimen examples because they contained no wisdom. (I am indebted to McMullin, 1967, for the gist of this summary).

An early turn toward empiricist science can be found in Newton, who "combined a Galilean stress on exact mathematically expressed data with a Baconian stress on observation and constant progressive testing. Newton emphasized the observational origin of his specific mechanical laws (like those governing gravitational or rotational motions) in a way Galileo had not; he emphasized the importance of a quantitative structuring of experience in a way Bacon had not" (McMullin, 1967, p. 366). On the other hand, Newton also practiced alchemy, and there is reason to believe that his concept of gravity, made up of the forces of attraction and repulsion between particles of matter, may have been inspired in part by his knowledge of the occult (see Westfall, 1984, pp. 315–335). As a result of his fascination with some strands of conceptualist thinking, Newton was probably not the empiricist he claimed to be, and "in some important respects he not only departed from the narrow correlationism he liked to preach but even exhibited an assurance about the ultimacy of the basic concepts of his mechanics that was more than a little reminiscent of his great rationalist adversary, Descartes" (McMullin, 1967, p. 366).

Newton's followers showed a similar mixture of views. Following his death, the study of physics (and especially mechanics) became more generally empirical. But although Newton and Galileo are credited with creating the scientific revolution, they did not simultaneously mark the end of one era and the beginning of another. Just as traces of alchemy could be found in the work of well-known scientists throughout this middle period, so we can trace a mixture of conceptualist and empiricist views of the world into the middle of the nineteenth century (see Vickers, 1984). Freud came to science just as our modern empiricist view of it was beginning to hold sway, although conceptualism was by no means a dead subject. How does he fit into this background and what factors influenced him to play down his more respectable empirical heritage?

We have already noted the contrast between the classical nature of Freud's early experimental work and his mode of argument in *Die Traumdeutung*. Thanks to an illuminating paper by John Toews, we are now able to pinpoint almost precisely the moment in Freud's career when he moved from one type of science to another. This moment occurred shortly after he made public his well-known seduction theory to account for adult neurosis. Although his new account was "defiantly scandalous, tracing the suffering of the younger generation to the secret sexual perversions of their hypocritical elders . . . Freud also clearly believed that his theory was constructed and articulated within the context of a code of logical and empirical procedures that he shared with his enemies and doubters" (Toews, 1991, p. 509). But the discovery, as we have seen, was short-lived; in the famous letter to Fleiss, Freud was forced to admit that "I no longer believe in my *neurotica*." Only a year and a half after he had publicly announced an inductively grounded explanation, he began to realize that much of the evidence on which his reasoning had been based was more fantasy than reality; the data that had seemed so predictive now seemed open to other interpretations. As the importance of psychic reality became clearer in the etiology of neurosis, it raised the question whether this new kind of data could be extracted and evaluated according to classical Galilean methods. Freud may also have wondered whether the strict laws of inductive logic (which he had learned from a careful reading and translation of John Stuart Mill) continued to apply to unconscious modes of thought.

Toews summarizes his dilemma:

> The collapse of the seduction theory in the fall of 1897 was marked by a collapse of Freud's confidence in his ability to integrate fantasy-life into the project of reconstructing the real history of event sequences. Unable to differentiate fact from fiction in his patients' reports, he felt the reality reference of his investigation dissolving under his feet. (p. 513)

Since the determining events were often outside the patient's awareness, Freud realized that a new methodology, resting on a new species of reasoning, was required. His first attempts in this direction make up *Die Traumdeutung* and his account of the Dora case. He never again attempted to reason in strict inductive fashion from a series of cases, and from this time on seemed more comfortable within the Aristotelian tradition.

There are at least four other factors that seem to have played a role in this paradigm shift. First and foremost, as we have seen in the preceding chapter, there was the influence of immediate circumstances on Freud's conclusions. If largely personal reasons forced him to reconsider his conclusions, it was much easier to resort to prescientific methods to justify his new approach; he could hardly point to a public data base when the evidence was private.

Second, there was Freud's friendship with Fliess. During the time he was grappling with his new awareness of fantasy as a determining factor in the patient's illness, Freud's relationship with Fliess began to cool. The relationship was particularly threatened by the Emma Eckstein scandal, when Fliess bungled a nose operation on a patient initially referred by Freud, a mistake that almost resulted in death from a serious loss of blood. The near-fatal disaster might easily have shaken Freud's faith in his colleague and removed some of the aura surrounding Fliess's bio-mathematical theories, which were seemingly grounded on a secure empirical base. If this example of empirical reasoning could entail such an obvious clinical failure, then Freud may have had additional doubts about the wisdom of a strictly Galilean approach in his own upcoming investigations. As his relationship to

Fliess began to cool, he may also have reduced his identification with the nineteenth-century positivistic tradition. (See Toews, 1991, and Sulloway, 1979, for a more extended discussion of the Freud-Fliess friendship and its bearing on Freud's methodology).

A third influence on Freud's view of science was his own developing self-analysis. Toews's description best presents the case: As he became "the theoretical possessor not only of his own case history but also of his own scientific realm—the inner reality of unconscious psychic life (the body as lived from the inside) which was equal in status to the external biological reality that was Fliess' domain—[he could] assume the position of ancestor rather than heir, father rather than son" (1991, p. 520). Although the importance of the self-analysis can also be overestimated, as we will see in Chapter 5, its discoveries gave Freud a set of clinical data that Fliess had no way of explaining.

Finally, there is the possibility of what might be called a case of associative learning. It was the inductive tradition that led directly to Freud's seduction hypothesis and the triumphant announcement of his discovery. When only months later he was forced to retract his revolutionary theory, we can speculate that some of the surrounding embarrassment may have rubbed off on his attitude toward the Galilean paradigm. Shaken by this loss of face, Freud may have placed some of the blame on his overreliance on classical empiricist methodology and, as a consequence, renewed his efforts to find a more useful alternative.

But it should not be assumed that Freud closed the door once and for all on the classical Galilean approach. As late as 1915, he was celebrating the virtues of inductive reasoning by pointing to the importance of beginning with a series of clinical observations that are gradually organized into more abstract ideas by means of tentative and indefinite suppositions—a kind of scaffolding laid over the building under construction. The separate parts of this scaffolding "are in the nature of conventions—although everything depends on their not being arbitrarily chosen but determined by their having significant relations to the empirical material, relations that we seem to sense before we can clearly recognize and demonstrate them. It is only after more thorough investigation of the field of observation that we are able to formulate its basic scientific concepts with increased precision, and progressively so to modify them that they become serviceable and consistent over a wide area" (1915, p. 117). But while he may have argued on behalf of the standard methodology, the manner in which he actually dealt with his data tells quite a different story.

Die Traumdeutung brings us his first collection of dream examples, his initial data base. If he were to continue in an empiricist tradition, Freud would next attempt to reduce these examples to a small number of general principles that would then be applied—in a crucial next step—to a new set of dream specimens. Following the advice of Robert Boyle, he should set himself "diligently and industriously to make experiments and collect observations, without being overforward to establish principles and axioms, believing it uneasy to erect such theories as are capable to explicate all the phenomena of nature before they have taken notice of a tenth part of those phenomena that are to be explicated" (cited in McMullin, 1967, p. 354).

Freud never carries out this assignment. Although *Die Traumdeutung* goes through many editions, the set of dream specimens remains essentially the same. He goes partway toward deriving a set of principles from his first sample of observations—we can think of his assertion that an infantile wish is a necessary cause of any dream, regardless of content, and his distinction between the secondary process, the basis for normal waking thought, and the primary process, which forms the basis for dream thinking. But he never takes the important step of gathering a new set of specimens. Instead of adopting a conventional empiricist approach to the understanding of dreams, Freud seems to fall back on the older, conceptualist approach. He takes refuge in a cherished set of examples—his dream specimens—and depends on their plausibility to sustain his argument. He urges the reader to follow his reasoning, to become familiar with his network of associations, and in this way, to come to appreciate his insight. This approach contrasts with that of Newton, some two hundred years earlier:

> For Newton, the primary warrant of a scientific claim was the set of experimental data that one could bring in its support. It was not its self-evidence; he realized that his theory of colors, for example, had no sort of intrinsic conceptual necessity about it and had to be derived from a finite and specially designed set of experiments . . . The grounds for his theories of gravitation and of dispersion did not lie in an insight into their conceptual necessity nor in their coherence

as an explanatory causal structure. Rather, it was the way in which they accounted exactly for the mathematically expressed data of observation. (McMullin, 1967, p. 363)

Freud tended to place more emphasis on the self-evident quality of a set of associations and the link between dream and associations. In the last resort, he would appeal to his private clinical experience. This kind of argument is clearly conceptualist, not empiricist, because it claims a special privilege for the investigator, who, because of special insights, particular experiences, or special training, has a clearer view of the phenomenon in question. This special position makes certain conclusions self-evident (at least to him). It was assumed that the "human mind has a quality of 'insight' . . . which allows it to grasp essence via single observations. It is this power of seeing the universal in the singular that makes the premises of natural science into necessary truths that are *seen* to be such, without the need for further test" (McMullin, 1967, p. 337). Since the truth is known immediately, there is no point in collecting further examples; all that remains undone is to convince others. Persuasion comes about by the careful study of the core specimens, which must be continued until the reader comes to understand Freud's conclusions.

We can see how a conceptualist theory of science leads directly to the master-apprentice tradition, a central part of psychoanalytic training; to a relaxed attitude toward gathering new observations and toward the general principle of hypothesis-testing; to an impatience with alternative points of view (the truth is largely known); and above all, to a fascination with the original collection of core examples—the dream specimens. This collection, judged self-evident by Freud who saw no need to make extensive revisions in subsequent editions of *Die Traumdeutung,* is supposed to contain the essence of our wisdom, and its full store of riches is still to be mined. Our task is to devote ourselves to the painstaking study of the most important dreams, collect all possible information about the conditions under which they were dreamt (see Grinstein, 1983), and in every way possible, put ourselves into Freud's shoes. Then—and only then—will we understand his findings.

The extent to which psychoanalytic teaching is still grounded in Freud's specimen dreams and five classic cases can be taken as a mark of its Aristotelian (conceptualist) heritage. To the extent that original specimens are still taught in psychoanalytic institutes as the essential source of knowledge to be passed on, item by item and case by case, to each new generation of candidates—to that extent, we must conclude that psychoanalysis is as much a medieval as a modern science. Whether Freud was brought to this position by the influence of Franz Brentano (a specialist on Aristotle with whom he took five philosophy courses [see Ramzy, 1956, and Sulloway, 1979, p. 92, n.27]), or whether the form of the material dictated the solution, it seems important to realize the depth and breadth of the Aristotelian heritage of psychoanalysis and how far it still deviates from contemporary, empirical science. This heritage has important implications for an understanding of the special significance of the *Standard Edition,* for a sharper awareness of the relation between evidence and theory, and for a resolution of the current hermeneutic debate, because it can be argued that conceptualist science has many hermeneutic features. We may finally agree that psychoanalysis is a science—but a science of a very special kind.

3 Aristotelian and Medieval Influences

We have seen the importance of the specimen in *Die Traumdeutung* and in the clinical literature in general (the clinician's fascination with the single case reflects the teachings of Aristotelian science). According to these assumptions, one good example was worth a thousand bad ones, and once a good specimen had been discovered, there was no need to search for further instantiations of the rule. The sufficiency of the good example helps to explain why Freud never revised his dream book in any radical manner; it also helps to account for the almost sacred nature of the favorite specimen—dream, presenting symptom, or case study—in the psychoanalytic literature. Because it contained a near-infinite array of wisdom, it was thought to deserve the careful attention of successive generations of scholars, each new wave building on the findings of the one before, always assuming that something more remained to be discovered.

This fascination with the single specimen and the belief that its secrets can never be exhausted provides a striking contrast with Galilean science. For the post-Renaissance investigator, examples were expendable and more-or-less equivalent, one being no better than another. It was an apple falling from an apple tree that supposedly inspired Newton to develop his theory of gravitation, but we have no interest in knowing what kind of apple; there is no attempt, in this or similar cases, to document the original specimen and protect it for posterity. In like fashion, the objects Galileo supposedly dropped from the Leaning Tower are not preserved in a vacuum case in some scientific Hall of Fame. These objects only serve to instantiate the general rule—that "falling objects of different weights fall with equal velocities and with a uniform acceleration." It is because the axiom brooks

48

no exceptions that the examples are interchangeable and essentially uninteresting in themselves. By contrast, in Aristotelian science, the general principle, never very powerful, always gave way to the individual case.

The complexity of the chosen specimen goes hand in hand with the fact that no two specimens are interchangeable. This complexity gave rise to the fascination with the individual specimen; because it could not be reduced to a general rule, it stimulated multiple attempts to understand and uncover its true essence. "All phenomena," writes Reiss, "are thus subject to an unlimited series of interpretations, and any 'explanation' [is subject] to a limitless series of variations" (1982, p. 142). In his attempt to understand each specimen in all its many aspects and within a range of different contexts, the medieval scientist was not attempting to reduce the case to a single rule (such as the law of gravitation). Partly for this reason, specimens were never interchangeable.

When the psychoanalyst returns once again (as he still does) to the Irma dream in order to study some new aspect against a new context, or when he celebrates a new telling of the self-analysis legend (as in Gay, 1988), or when he begins a new reading of the Dora case, either from a feminist perspective or from some other vantage point—in all of these activities, he is underscoring his fascination with the specimen and repeating his belief in its capacity to teach him something never found before. It is partly because the specimen cannot be reduced to a formula or law that its essence can only be revealed by a thorough study of its complexity; and because its complexity defies a single inspection, repeated scrutiny is the only solution.

Because the specimen is sacred, it matters most; the specimen counts over the investigator and over the method. Once again, we might note the contrast with Galilean science, in which examples are expendable and the investigator (and to a lesser extent, the method) take all the credit. It was the (lowercase) apple that inspired (uppercase) Newton to discover the law of gravity; empiricist science celebrates the individual, not the example. Aristotelian science, in putting the specimen before the investigator, takes the position that "God is in the details" and that "Nature is not only stranger than we imagine; it is stranger than we can possibly imagine" (Haldane; cited in Tracy, 1981, p. 359).

Let us now consider the assumptions of Aristotelian science from a more general perspective, paying particular attention to four important features (Lewin, 1931, McMullin, 1967, and Vickers, 1984, provide more extended descriptions of the contrast between Aristotelian and Galilean modes of thought).

First, the medieval scientist believed that only certain parts of the natural world possessed a completely predictable structure. "For Aristotle, those things are lawful, conceptually intelligible, which occur *without exception* [and] . . . which occur *frequently* . . . In other words, the ambition of science to understand the complex, chaotic, and unintelligible world, its faith in the ultimate decipherability of this world, was limited to such events as were *certified* by repetition in the course of history to possess a certain persistence and stability" (Lewin, 1931, pp. 144–145). The importance of repetition applied to the display of naturally occurring events, such as sunrise and sunset, the tides, the seasons, and—for the physician—the symptoms and syndromes of illness. Repetition in nature was to be distinguished from repetition by experiment; the first was an Aristotelian principle; the second would become a Galilean mode of thought. For Aristotle, the concept of lawfulness was primarily historic: "stress was laid not upon the 'general validity' which modern physics understands by lawfulness, but upon the events in the historically given world which displayed the required stability. The highest degree of lawfulness, beyond mere frequency, was characterized by the idea of the always eternal" (Lewin, 1931, p. 147).

Because "class membership defined the essence or essential nature of the object" (Lewin, 1931, p. 143), the individual case that belonged to a regularly occurring class of events could be defined as the prototype of that class. Such objects seemed particularly appropriate as specimens for more detailed study because it was assumed that they contained all the important features of the class; thus a carefully chosen single case could be used to answer a wide range of general questions. The one-of-a-kind event, on the other hand, was felt to be of little conceptual interest: the "individual event seems . . . fortuitous, unimportant, scientifically indifferent" (Lewin, 1931, p. 151).

All aspects of the chosen specimen were deemed worthy of systematic examination. Toward the end of the Middle Ages, thoughtful investigators were told that "fresh observations of nature should form the basis of a new science" (Debus, 1965, p. 14). Followers of the new movement were told to sell your lands, your houses, your clothes and your jewelry; burn up your books. On the other hand ... note with care the distinctions between animals, the difference of plants, the various kinds of minerals, the *property and origins of everything that exists.* (Severinus, 1571; cited in Debus, 1965, p. 20; italics mine)

The specimen object was thought to be the supreme source of knowledge, and all questions were to be settled by a close inspection of the chosen case:

Some students asked Vesalius [around 1540] what the true fact about these movements was, whether the arteries followed the movement of the heart, or whether they had a movement different from the heart. Vesalius answered: "I do not want to give you my opinion, please *feel for yourselves with your own hands and trust them."* (Ruben Erikkson, 1959; cited in Bylebyl, 1985, p. 235; italics mine)

Once the specimen had been discovered (or decided upon), attention turned to a close inspection of all its apparent and concealed attributes.

Second, it was assumed that the essence of the specimen object was essentially transparent to the inquiring scientist. Some specimens required extended study, but others were immediately transparent and revealed their meaning in a single observation:

The dissection of a live animal will teach anyone that when the heart contracts, blood is poured forth from the left ventricle into the aorta, whence it seems necessary for the aorta to dilate; but when the heart dilates the aorta contracts. (Casper Bauhim, 1597; cited in Bylebyl, 1985, p. 238)

In either case, their contents were revealed only to the qualified observer. "It is this power of seeing the universal in the singular," writes McMullin, "that makes the premises of natural science into necessary truths that are *seen* to be such, without the need for further test" (1967, p. 337). In contrast to the science of Bacon and the Royal Society, which emphasized the democratic character of discovery, open to any participating observer, Aristotelian science was a much more elitist affair and true insight into nature was thought to be the privilege of the naturally gifted observer.

The so-called transparency of the object was closely connected to a failure to distinguish phenotype from genotype (see Lewin, 1931). The Aristotelian scientist believed that the analysis of surface features exhausted the properties of the object. He had no notion of the possibility that differently appearing objects might be similar in some deeper sense, or that regularity might be discovered over long periods when it did not appear in smaller samples. Only a Galilean scientist could recognize, for example, that the same law (gravity) applies to stones thrown off a tower and to planets revolving around the sun.

Third, it was assumed that if immediate understanding of the target specimen was not forthcoming, it would appear sooner or later. The Aristotelian scientist thus assumed a largely passive stance in his quest for knowledge and waited for inspiration to strike and reveal the nature of the target object. Galilean scientists, by contrast, used the experiment as their primary tool and depended on controlled manipulation of the variables to enable them to discover the secrets of Nature.

Fourth, the Aristotelian scientist assumed what might be called an *analogue* view of the world (see Spence, 1973, for a general statement of the analogue-digital distinction). Explanation was grounded in similarity and difference; the nature of the target object was partly determined by finding the ways in which it corresponded to other, better-studied aspects of nature. By contrast, the Galilean scientist tried whenever possible to quantify his observations, thus taking a *digital* approach to the world. Quantification grew naturally out of experimentation and allowed him not only to share his findings more easily with his colleagues and evaluate attempts at replication more precisely, but gradually, as the principles of probability were better understood, to more accurately measure the significance of his results. The digital approach was closely correlated with the emerging emphasis on general laws and the decline of interest in the single specimen.

When Freud announced the conclusions of his seduction theory, he rested his case on eighteen accounts that seemed to make up a homogeneous series and support a single conclusion. After he realized that he was basing his theory on a mixture of fact and fantasy, he may have concluded that in this new science, a superficial similarity among cases was no longer a sufficient basis for argument. Because the inductive tradition tempted the investigator to focus more on the size of the sample than on the individual instance, it might have seemed to Freud to be more misleading than helpful. Further study of the clinical examples made it clear that surface did not always correspond to depth, and if surface was untrustworthy, then a science grounded on the similarity of surface features could only be misleading.

But in retreating to the individual specimen for his understanding of the larger phenomenon, Freud replaced one kind of error with another. Aristotelians defended the detailed study of the target object on the grounds that it synthesized all the important features of the larger class, and they were understandably dubious about the exceptional case. But Freud's so-called specimen dreams are more exceptions than true specimens; they are, after all, one-time occurrences that carry enormous significance for him but can hardly be described as representative examples of a larger class (except for certain interesting exceptions such as the examination dream, which turns out to have a general lawfulness that is not specific to circumstances or dreamer). It is tempting to argue that it was their personal meaningfulness which fooled him into believing that they were scientifically meaningful as well.

Once he had given up the attempt to follow an inductive line of reasoning and look beyond the single specimen, Freud was never able to separate *necessary* and *contingent* features of the final explanation. The interpretation of the Irma dream, for example, is probably some combination of both necessary and contingent features, but so long as we only have one dream of this kind, we can never separate the two categories. It was partly the awareness of this confusion during the Renaissance that led to the gradual abandonment of the Aristotelian approach to explanation and helped to bring about an increasing reliance on the inductive method. One specimen, it was felt, no matter how carefully examined and rigorously restudied, might still contain features that were irrelevant to the final description. Some aspects of the chosen specimen might co-occur simply because of gratuitous features of that particular example; to make these aspects the ingredients of the final explanation was to confuse necessary and contingent features of the specimen and hopelessly confound the final explanation. The accepted description (and, therefore, the explanation) of the chosen specimen might often represent possible rather than fundamental relationships between the chosen parts. Precisely because there were no *a priori* grounds for selection of the specimen, the investigator was always at the mercy of circumstance.

One virtue of the inductive method stems from the fact that if enough samples are examined, the contingent features tend to cancel each other out, and what is left—the common denominator of the series—tends to be the necessary core of the explanation. The larger the range of observations, the more certainty we attach to the result.

This conclusion is grounded in Hume's Principle of the Uniformity of Nature, which asserts that "the observation of past regularities gives us grounds for predicting that the same regularities will recur in the future" (Kukla, 1989, p. 791).

Had Freud gone ahead with his original intention and collected a second set of dreams to confirm his initial observations, he would have minimized the role of contingent features in his explanation and arrived at a more general theory of dreaming. It can even be argued that his account of the examination dream follows a more inductive tradition; in this case, he was able to abstract the general features of these dreams, and his account still stands. But his explanation of the more famous specimen dreams suffers from the very fact that makes them fascinating—the particularities of the event get in the way of a more general explanation, and it could be argued that it was the fascination with the specific that prevented Freud from seeing the error of his ways.

The Doctrine of Signatures

It is a matter of record that Freud studied with Franz Brentano, and thus it should not be surprising to find him tempted by certain aspects of the Aristotelian tradition. But much more troubling than the fondness for specimen cases is the evidence in psychoanalytic thinking of a worldview that had been popular before the Renaissance but was more or less discredited by the Baconian Revolution. This view, called the *doctrine of signatures,* was grounded in the belief that the "nature of things, their co-existence, the way in which they are linked together and communicate, is nothing other than their resemblance. And that resemblance is visible only in the network of signs that crosses the world from one end to the other" (Foucault, 1973, p. 29). The medieval scientist looked on the world as a system of signatures—the outward sign of a buried similarity. The signature was not a direct copy of the object's essence but represented a certain kind of transformation. The skilled investigator of the natural world was familiar with all forms of transformation and was practiced at discovering the signature even when it was heavily disguised. This fascination with the signature was directly connected with a failure to appreciate extreme phenotype-genotype discontinuities.

It is of more than passing interest to find Freud applying a kind of signature analysis to the interpretation of dreams and symptoms. The latent dream thought or underlying conflict is assumed to be transformed, by one or more primary process mechanisms, into its manifest content. Understanding comes about by reversing the process. In full agreement with the theory of signatures, the dream interpreter solves the dream ("detects its signature") by selecting the right mechanism of transformation, applying it to the manifest dream, and discovering the essence of the latent dream.

The search for hidden signs has become an essential part of the general psychoanalytic approach to meanings. A budding amaryllis bulb with its long stalk and emerging head strikes us immediately as phallic; the speaker who suddenly loses his voice we describe as castrated. The world of natural objects has become, once again, a world of hidden and not-so-hidden meanings, opaque to the naive but transparent to the initiated, who see below the surface into the depths of being. The spread of psychoanalytic theory has brought us back to the Middle Ages once again. We search the world for resemblances that will tell us what latent content lies beneath the surface appearance. We may not believe (as did Paracelsus) that it is God's will to allow "nothing to remain without exterior and visible signs in the form of special marks—just as a man who has buried a hoard of treasure marks the spot that he may find it again" (quoted in Foucault, 1973, p. 26)—but we still believe that psychoanalysis has made us better readers of the text of the world and that ever since Freud, we see further and deeper into the surface of things. But in adopting this approach, we are not significantly different from the scientists at the end of the sixteenth century who believed that "resemblance played a constructive role in the knowledge of Western culture. It was resemblance that largely guided exegesis and the interpretation of texts; it was resemblance that organized the play of symbols, made possible knowledge of things visible and invisible, and controlled the art of representing them" (Foucault, 1973, p. 17).

The psychoanalyst not only sees the world as a collection of symbols ("signatures") waiting to be deciphered, he also listens to language with an ear tuned to slips, neologisms, and other speech faults, which provide clues to disguised meaning. A speech fault is never accidental or happenstance; it is every bit as indicative as any classical signature, and its presence is meant to be noted and deciphered. We also share the medieval belief that "the world is covered with signs that must be deciphered, and those signs, which reveal resemblances and affinities, are themselves no more than forms of similitude. To know must therefore be to interpret: to find a way from the visible mark to that which is being said by it and which, without that mark, would lie like unspoken speech, dormant within things" (Foucault, 1973, p. 32).

Knowledge, in short, flows from interpretation, and there is no limit to what can be known, what new signatures can be decoded. But it should be noted that this knowledge lies in the world and cannot be separated from it; it cannot be catalogued, abstracted, or argued over because the wisdom is contained in the particular specimen, and while the specimen may produce insight of a particular kind, we have no way of representing this insight apart from its vehicle. We see this problem in the extended analyses of Freud's specimen dream. The insights revealed in his gloss of the Irma dream contribute to our general fund of knowledge, but they cannot be reduced to a set of principles or replicated by the discoveries gained from other dreams. In similar fashion, medieval knowledge also consisted of long lists, many of them secret and known only to circles of initiates or members of occult orders. Because this knowledge could not be catalogued or hierarchically arranged, it could only be learned by rote, example after example, concept after concept. While followers of the theory of signatures believed the world to be ultimately transparent, they also had to believe that the knowledge base to be derived from this world must be no smaller than the world itself (see Foucault, 1973, pp. 30–34).

The wisdom of *Die Traumdeutung* is essentially contained in the dreams themselves and in Freud's commentaries on them. In similar fashion, the insights revealed by a study of Freud's five cases cannot be separated from the cases themselves. We now begin to realize why such special significance attaches to *Die Traumdeutung* and the five cases. Their wisdom is essentially interpretative and comes only from a close reading of the clinical text, which entails a search for its signatures and their hidden meaning.

The doctrine of signatures represented an essential part of the occult tradition that flourished up to the time of the Renaissance. The natural world was felt to be important not for what it seemed to be but for what it concealed by way of hidden messages from God. Correspondence was assumed to exist between the natural world and the heavenly bodies (as in astrology). More particularly, it was thought that there was a connection between the universe, or Macrocosm, and the individual, or Microcosm. This connection was particularly important in medicine; doctors were advised to study the influence of the moon, the planets, and the stars on the course of illness. Certain illnesses were explained in terms of their correspondence to macroscopic phenomena; thus apoplexy was thought to be analogous to a thunderstorm and treatment was guided by this similarity. As a general rule, it was thought that "to understand and explain anything consisted for a thinker of this time in showing that it was not what it appeared to be, but that it was the symbol or sign of a more profound reality, that it proclaimed or signified something else" (Gilson; cited in Crombie, 1979, vol. 1, p. 37).

How was this task accomplished? The medieval scientist considered himself a master at detecting the hidden "signature" that would reveal the object's true nature (its essence). Skill at detecting the object's essence was based on the ability to map out what Foucault (1973) has called "the paths of similitude and . . . the directions they take." Clues to these connections "must be indicated on the surface of things; there must be visible marks for the invisible analogies" (p. 26). To the initiated, "the face of the world is covered with blazons, with characters, with ciphers and obscure words . . . the space inhabited by immediate resemblances becomes like a vast open book; it bristles with written signs" (p. 27). As I have already noted, the modern psychoanalyst works in much the same manner, constantly searching for resemblances and pattern matches and using standard transformations to bridge the gap between two apparently dissimilar examples.

The search for essences during the Middle Ages would typically begin by first singling out a category for investigation. The scientist would choose from one of Aristotle's ten categories of Substance, Quantity, Quality, Relation, Place, Time, Posture, State, Action, and Passion. To describe (and ultimately explain) a pen, for example, the scientist would observe that it was "long and thin, that it is black, that it is mine, that it is resting on the point of its nib, on this piece of paper, at 9 p.m., that it is filled with ink, that it makes a blue mark, and that it is being held by hand" (Southern, 1953, p. 180). The ten categories were thought to exhaust the properties of the object.

Once the category had been established, the next job was to establish the true essence of the object. If it was not apparent from an inspection of its class membership (by looking, for example, at a sequence of observations), the investigator would use his intuition to identify the underlying signature and then, by making use of one of the four similitudes, find a link between surface appearance and underlying content. Reasoning of this kind depended on the use of established principles of transformation. It was by the application of these principles that one could decide whether two appearances were the same or different. "It was resemblance that largely guided exegesis and the interpretation of texts; it was resemblance that organized the play of symbols, made possible knowledge of things visible and invisible, and controlled the art of representing them" (Foucault, 1973, p. 17). The four similitudes can be defined (drawing heavily on Foucault) as follows:

1. *Convenientia* calls our attention to contiguity and teaches us that forms that appear in close proximity share a common feature. "In this hinge between things," writes Foucault, "a resemblance appears," and things that occur together tend to resemble one another. Body and soul, for example, are doubly convenient: the soul is influenced by the body, while the body is "altered and corrupted by the passions of the soul" (Porta, 1655; cited in Foucault, 1973, p. 18). Convenience varies with proximity; the closer together the target objects, the more features they have in common. "In the vast syntax of the world, the different beings adjust themselves to one another; the plant communicates with the animal, the earth with the sea, man with everything around him" (p. 18).

2. *Aemulatio* is a species of convenience that can function from a distance. "The human face, from afar, emulates the sky, and just as man's intellect is an imperfect reflection of God's wisdom, so his two eyes, with their limited brightness, are a reflection of the vast illumination spread across the sky by sun and moon" (p. 19). Because the connection is sustained through space, the similitude between members of the target pair may be more difficult to discover. "The stars," wrote Crollius (1624), "are the matrix of all plants and every star in the sky is only the spiritual prefiguration of a plant, such that it represents that plant, and just as each herb or plant is a terrestrial star looking up at the sky, so also each star is a celestial plant in spiritual form" (p. 20). We might here note the way in which microcosm is linked to macrocosm.

3. *Analogy* combined the two similitudes of convenience and emulation. "Like the latter, it makes possible the marvellous confrontation of resemblances across space; but it also speaks, like the former, of

adjacencies, of bonds and joints" (p. 21). Plants and animals are analogous because the vegetable can be thought of as an animal living head down with its mouth—or roots—buried in the earth; conversely, the plant can be thought of as an upright animal (see p. 21). By this reasoning, knowledge of plant nutrition and the role of roots and branches will help us understand the operation of veins and arteries and make us better able to cure the sick. Once an analogy was established, it was possible for medieval scientists to use the first member of the pair as a guide to understanding the second. Because man was thought to be an analogy for the universe (substituting microcosm for macrocosm), the description (and explanation) of apoplexy was grounded in the observation of a tempest: "The storm begins when the air becomes heavy and agitated, the apoplectic attack at the moment when our thoughts become heavy and disturbed; then the clouds pile up, the belly swells, the thunder explodes and the bladder bursts; the lightning flashes and the eyes glitter with a terrible brightness, the rain falls, the mouth foams, the thunderbolt is unleashed and the spirits burst open breaches in the skin, but then the sky becomes clear again, and in the sick man reason regains ascendancy [the storm passes]" (p. 23).

4. *Sympathy*, the final similitude, requires no grounds of similarity between the target pairs; it is the freest of all the principles and therefore the most arbitrary. Sympathy explains why fire, because it is warm and light, rises into the air (which is also light); it explains why the sunflower (which is yellow) turns toward the sun (which is also yellow). But sympathy can also be determined by history alone; thus the roses at a funeral will acquire the mood of the ceremony and their blossoms will fall prematurely because they are "in mourning." Free to operate across space and time, sympathy is the most powerful of all the similitudes and the hardest to identify.

Access to the four similitudes gave the medieval scientist the key to understanding the world by going from surface to depth and vice versa. The target object—a sunflower, a wilting rose, or an attack of apoplexy—was first searched for the presence of the signature, the outward sign of a buried similarity. Once the appropriate signature had been identified, it was then possible to determine which of the four similitudes had been at work; by reasoning backward, the scientist could then determine the essence of the target object. Explanation (and treatment) followed directly from description. If apoplexy was similar (through analogy) to a thunderstorm, then it followed that its course was short-lived and it would leave no permanent effects. It can be seen that a well-chosen analogy could function as a kind of medieval Merck Manual; the more compelling the analogy, the more it explained and the more it contributed to the fame of its originator. Much of the reputation of Paracelsus, the noted medieval physician, stemmed from his eye for apt analogies. With Paracelsus, writes Tempkin, "the analogy almost takes the place of the parable in the New Testament. To make the reader see the truth of his interpretation, Paracelsus has no other means but to lead him as near as possible through examples . . . These pictures, these visions are offered as interpretations of what is otherwise hidden and obscure in its cause" (1952, p. 211).

Extended knowledge of the ten categories and the four similitudes, together with experience in their application, allowed the medieval scientist to connect everything with everything else. Explanation followed from classification because causal analysis followed directly from description. But the basis for these explanations was the surface features of the objects in question; as a result, it became more difficult to group together what was manifestly dissimilar. This focus on surface attributes forced the medieval scientist to put into separate classes the "orbits of the planets, the oscillation of a pendulum" (Lewin, 1931, p. 149) even though we now know that each of these examples is an expression of the same underlying principle: the law of gravity. Thus the emphasis on surface features tended to conceal the importance of underlying themes that might assume different forms. Here, once again, we see a failure to appreciate the phenotype-genotype distinction.

A second problem stemmed from the open nature of the analytic system. A little thought will show that the search for the revealing signature can easily become highly arbitrary (and I will have more to say about this problem later). When studying a sunflower, do we focus on its color (which leads us to find, through *sympathy*, its similitude with the sun) or on its membership in the plant family (which leads us to think, through *analogy*, of its similitude to man)? With no obvious grounds for deciding on either signature or similitude, it can be seen that experience, authority, and tradition could take the place of observation. Felicitous analogies, functioning like parables, could stand in the way of further investigation. The very flexibility of analogic reasoning generated (and guaranteed) an explanation for everything, but the explanation was judged more on aesthetic than scientific grounds, and if it was found compelling, it quickly became rooted in tradition. Pleasing explanations then became the barrier to better explanations.

Similitudes in Clinical Practice

Each of the classical similitudes has a parallel in current psychoanalytic practice. The emphasis on contiguity found in *convenientia* is expressed in the analyst's sensitivity to the sequence of associations; it is widely assumed that if thought B follows thought A during a sequence of associations, then A is the cause of B. If an interpretation, to take another example, is followed by a new memory, it is assumed that the latter was caused by the former, and that close inspection of the memory will reveal a way in which it represents one or more aspects of the interpretation. The search for resemblance between these two expressions, although phrased in different language, is an application of the similitude of *convenientia*. This similitude also comes into play when associations that follow a dream are assumed to be about the dream, even though the connection is not indicated by the patient; once again, contiguity alerts the clinician to a possible connection. It is also assumed, as with the similitude, that resemblance varies directly with proximity; the closer the target objects are together, the more they have in common.

Turning to the second similitude, we can find examples of *aemulatio* in almost every pattern match that is not governed by contiguity. An obvious example presents itself in the analysis of transference. The analyst is trained to be particularly sensitive to resemblances between interactions within the hour and significant events in the outside world. The detection and interpretation of transference can be seen as an application of *aemulatio,* because the pattern match may be traced across changes in space and time as well as across other transformations (such as gender). Detection of so-called derivatives provides another class of pattern matches based on *aemulatio*. Suppose the patient is expecting to terminate her therapy in three-weeks time and finds herself aggressively cleaning out, dusting, and repainting a walk-in closet. By raising the question "Why now?," the analyst is able to point to a link between the end of therapy and the housecleaning, and in this way, show the patient that the activity can be seen as a derivative of the termination. Both activities represent the end of one phase of her life and the beginning of another. Further links might be discovered between closet (a walk-in closet with no windows) and her mind, and between psychoanalysis and housecleaning (it will be recalled that Freud referred to free associations as "chimney sweepings").

Clues to this kind of pattern match are often contained in their timing, and Time, as I have noted, is one of Aristotle's ten categories. The analyst might begin by noting that two apparently dissimilar events took place at roughly the same time. This seeming coincidence alerts him to the possibility that they may have something in common, and he explores the likelihood of a soft pattern match, using the transformation of *aemulatio*. Choice of category comes first, to be followed by choice of similitude and then a detailed exploration of the pattern match. We will find this sequence repeated in many of the clinical examples detailed below. To the extent that it represents a typical form of clinical reasoning, it gives us one more reason to understand how medieval forms of thinking are particularly relevant to the art and science of interpretation in clinical psychoanalysis.

The last example can also be used to illustrate the application of *analogy,* the third classical similitude. To the extent that the activity of cleaning out the closet is a metaphor for the process of free association, we have further reason to believe that the first activity stands for the second. Further parallels may be seen between the design of a walk-in closet and the inaccessible nature of the unconscious: both locations are characterized by darkness and disarray. To extend the metaphor even further, it can be argued that cleaning out and repainting the closet is similar in many respects to the aims of therapy, an activity intended to restructure and refurbish the mind.

The use of *analogy* is restricted only by the limitations of the analyst's command of metaphor, simile, and other ways of finding links between words. Sensitivity to this kind of similitude would seem to be reinforced by the analyst's rhetorical talents, and I will return to this issue in the next chapter when I look more closely at the rhetorical voice of psychoanalysis. Some knowledge of literature and critical theory would also seem useful, insofar as these fields help to heighten the analyst's awareness of allusions and the role they play in establishing similarity between two utterances. A detailed knowledge of art history is also an obvious asset for identifying pattern matches and discovering resemblances. Suppose the patient is about to terminate the treatment and finds herself thinking of the painting *Two Models in Omaha* by Philip Pearlstein. Knowledge of this artist's work would make the analyst remember that Pearlstein characteristically truncates the figures of his models with the frame of the painting. Aware of this tendency, the analyst might find himself wondering what other things were being "cut off" in the patient's life. This line of thought might raise the question of whether the treatment was being ended in somewhat arbitrary fashion and whether the termination was either premature in fact or was perceived so by the patient. In following this line of associations, clearly some knowledge of Pearlstein's work is a necessary precondition.

The application of *sympathy*, the fourth and last similitude, is best established by the discovery of a pattern match that does not depend on either contiguity, similarity, or analogy. Detection of this class of resemblances is clearly the strictest test of the good analyst because he is deprived of all the usual clues and must depend on such ineffable variables as "intuition" or "empathy." But as we have seen, it is precisely because they rely on few tangible clues that pattern matches of this kind are apt to be more fanciful than real, depending, in the last analysis, on empty argument, which pretends to discover similarity where none exists.

At this point it might be useful to present a series of clinical examples, taken from the recent literature, which illustrate how the analyst undertakes a pattern match. We will consider on what kinds of evidence he bases his decision, how the match can be classified (hard or soft), and how its truth can be determined. We will then discuss the principles that seem to underlie these matches and the ways in which they compare with the principles of medieval science.

Example 1

> I know a man ... who attempted to grapple in analysis with the question of why he was attracted only to blond women. "I suppose," he said to the analyst, "that it's because angels are blond, and princesses in fairy tales. Blondes are golden, they belong to the dominant ethnic type." "Nonsense," the analyst said. "That has nothing to do with it. You are attracted to blondes for quite a simple reason—they are furthest from the color of feces." (Broyard, 1989, p. 14)

The analyst begins by focusing on the target object (blondes), focusing further on the category of Quality (in this case, color) and excluding all other dimensions. He then invokes the medieval similitude of antipathy (the opposite of sympathy); the choice of this transformation rule enables him to search for opposites and he arrives at feces. The analyst either assumes or has evidence to believe that the patient is repelled by feces; if so, then the principle of antipathy would suggest that he is attracted by blondes. It can be seen that neither the choice of category nor the choice of similitude is fully justified by the vignette. If we give the analyst the benefit of the doubt in both cases, the reasoning is fairly straightforward and perhaps even replicable, but if other judges were given the same category and similitude, they might not arrive at the same interpretation.

Also worth noting is the certainty of the analyst. Once he has discovered the true essence of the target object (blondes = feces), then he feels secure about his explanation. We are reminded of the assumptions of conceptualist science: the warrant for the claim is the self-evidence of the statement. There is no need to look further.

Example 2

The patient dreams "that she was in a foreign country, possibly Mexico, crawling on hard ground strewn with emeralds and other precious stones." As she collected them, a godlike voice prohibited her from continuing. Much later in the treatment, the following interpretation was offered to her:

> The gems were a representation of her brilliant, infantile self that had remained unavailable (repressed) to her everyday self-experience. The god had disapproved of her gathering up these emeralds of her self. But without these (nuclear self) gems, she was (later) the dead Victorian woman in a casket . . . She had not been given enough of a sense of being loved, or of affirmation of the value of her self in her developing years by her self-absorbed mother or, later, by her more responsive but infantilizing and ultimately disappointing father. And, already vulnerable and prone to a depressive sense of loss, she lost the gems her experiences with [her father] had given her, the gems which . . . for a moment at least she imagined to be hers. (Goldberg, 1978; cited in Reed, 1987, p. 424)

The interpretation begins by isolating the precious gems as the target object. Next, attention is focused on the category of Quality (their value) and then on the meaning of their latent content: what do the precious gems represent? Apparently without benefit of associations, the analyst makes the assumption that they stand for something equivalently precious; in effect, he selects the similitude of *aemulatio*. Because of the patient's depressive sense of loss and in view of her strained relations with both parents, he decides that gems stand for early closeness with the father. Reed (pp. 424–427) criticizes the way in which interpretation proceeds without benefit of associations; to put this charge in slightly different language, we could say that both signature and category are arbitrarily chosen. If, for the sake of argument, the analyst had selected *antipathy,* he would assume that the gems represented the opposite of precious. Had he selected the category of Place (that is, Mexico), his associations might have turned to *The Treasure of the Sierra Madre* and to the themes of loss and foul play. As a final comment, we should note once again the certainty that accompanies the pattern match.

Example 3

> The patient was a forty-year-old man who had had a previous analysis. He began his treatment . . . by saying that he would like to postpone payment of [the analyst's] fees for several months so that he could make a down payment on some property at a resort. [The analyst] agreed to the arrangement, being "convinced" that the patient had "simply" begun his treatment with the hope that unlike his previous analysis this treatment would be for him rather than for the analyst. "Buying . . . the property [writes Kohut] reinstated a specific situation from his early life [in which] he could be unencumbered by the stifling restrictions [of his] . . . joyless, guilt-producing mother . . . [and] his self-absorbed, attention-demanding father . . . This analysis had to begin with a reinstatement of the one situation of his childhood in which his personality had been able to unfold . . . without the restrictions of his home." (Kohut, 1984, pp. 73–74; cited in Rubovits-Seitz, 1988, p. 952)

Attention is first focused on the property at the shore resort and the way it invokes in the patient the sense of freedom and lack of restraints. Such an analysis implies the categories of Quality, State, and Affection. To the extent that this property "reinstates a specific situation from [the patient's] early life," the analyst has invoked the similitude of *aemulatio* (again without benefit of associations). It can be seen that the choice of both category and similitude is entirely arbitrary; had other choices been made, the analyst would arrive at quite a different interpretation.

Example 4

The patient had complained, for as long as he could remember, of having a sensation as he was falling asleep that his face

> was being engulfed by a sticky mass. [This symptom] had subsided during his first analysis, but had never disappeared entirely . . . About a year into the reanalysis, following a confluence of dreams and experiences, [the analyst] interpreted the hypnagogic symptoms of engulfment by a sticky mass as a fear of and a wish for oral contact with the mother. The interpretation appealed immediately and the symptom disappeared, except for a few times in a minor form. (Johan, 1985, p. 188)

How can we understand the pattern match that connects the hypnagogic sensation of being engulfed by a sticky mass with the patient's ambivalent thoughts about his mother? The interpretation begins by focusing attention on the stickiness of the sensation; the analyst then searches for its repetition in some other part of the patient's fantasy life. This tactic almost necessarily forces the choice of *aemulatio* as the operative similitude. Once this choice has been made, the rest of the interpretation follows directly. Its effect on the patient is quite remarkable.

Critique of the Doctrine of Signatures

It can be seen from the examples presented that the choice of similitude will always determine the specific content of the pattern match, yet this choice is always arbitrary and often a matter of taste. In some of the examples the choice was made without benefit of the patient's associations; in other cases it seemed to stem directly from an *a priori* decision about categories and similitudes. The clinical evidence is almost never sufficient to make the reader feel that the interpretation offered was a *necessary* consequence of the attributes of the target symptom, and a skeptic might argue that all pattern matches were entirely arbitrary, subjective, and almost certainly capitalized on chance. If they succeeded in making a difference, as was the case with Example 4, the skeptic would simply reply that the consequences had nothing to do with the interpretation but resulted from some other factor as yet unexplored.

To raise questions about the validity of the single case brings us back, once again, to the critical distinction between necessary and contingent propositions. It has been customary to assume that the former are true (or false) in all possible worlds and that the latter are true in some possible worlds and false in some possible worlds (see Kukla, 1989, p. 791). This line of reasoning warns us that if we base our conclusions on a single specimen, we take the chance that they are based entirely on contingent features which may never occur a second time; in other words, the possible world is limited to one and only one case. It would seem that the truth value of most clinical interpretations is contingent rather than necessary; this does not make them less true to the moment at hand, but it clearly restricts their range of generalizability. If we keep this distinction in mind, we can see how clinical discoveries (contingent propositions) will almost never lead to covering laws (necessary propositions) and why it is so difficult to build a general theory of the mind from a series of specific clinical discoveries. It also helps to make clear why it is difficult, if not impossible, to replicate clinical findings outside of the consulting room. An interpretation might be true only in the possible world—a certain time in the analysis in which both patient and analyst were present—and be false in all other domains (including the world of the laboratory). The proposition might also be false in the world of the printed page because it is often impossible to reproduce all the contingent elements of the target situation. It is perhaps a result of this slippage that many clinical accounts seem unconvincing or only partial explanations: the printed report is simply not isomorphic with the original, clinical event, and what was true in the latter, because of its contingent nature, is not true in the former.

The distinction between necessary and contingent propositions also tells us something about the clinician's fondness for what seems, at first glance, to be an outdated form of reasoning. The doctrine of signatures was abandoned during the Renaissance, in part because it did not lead to the discovery of necessary truths that are, by definition, true in all possible worlds. But the clinician may not be interested in generating covering laws that apply to all patients; indeed, he most certainly cannot afford to search for propositions of this kind, because such a search would neglect the particular patient under his care and would force him to ignore the many contingent truths that come his way. It would seem precisely *because* the clinician needs to extract the most information from the single specimen that he tends to fall back on outmoded forms of reasoning and why the discipline of psychoanalysis has perfected an approach to the specimen that shows an uncanny resemblance to the medieval emphasis on category and similitude.

Consider the remarkable success of the interpretation in Example 4: once the pattern match was established, the symptom disappeared almost completely. Can we say that its effect is proof that the interpretation was correct? To answer yes would imply that the fantasy attributed to the patient—wanting and not wanting oral-vaginal contact with the mother—had actually been present at some time in his childhood. But the scope of the interpretation may, in fact, be much less general and may apply only to the specific moment of the single clinical session when the interpretation was first proposed. That moment constitutes the possible world in which the interpretation is true. In all other worlds, it may quite possibly be false. In other words, its remarkable success may depend on the full set of contingent features in that particular hour, which might include the patient's sense of being understood, the analyst's conviction (conveyed by his voice and phrasing) that he was correct, and what might be called the rhetorical demand of the moment: the possibility that some explanation was needed for the recurrent symptom and that the answer offered at that particular time happened to fill that need. But time and place are everything if the explanation is contingent. If it does not generalize beyond this particular here and now, then we cannot assume that we have discovered something of interest about the patient's fantasy life as a child. Nor can we assume that our theory of infantile development is in any way strengthened by the success of this interpretation, because such a theory presupposes the uncovering of a necessary (and therefore more general) truth.

We begin to see a conflict between the requirements of the clinician and the demands of normal, Galilean science. The former is particularly interested in the specific details of time and place; normal science, by contrast, is grounded on the use of the inductive method and the search for necessary truths, which, by definition, are assumed to hold true over the widest possible range of relevant domains. Because interpretations are always contingent and apply only to the specific situation, the clinician is almost always in error when he asserts a one-time observation as a general truth. At the same time, he is also prone to error if he relies too exclusively on the principles of normal science for the validation of general laws. Too faithful a devotion to the general will cause him to lose sight of the particular.

It seems clear that the clinician's primary motive is to make maximal sense of the clinical material, which means, in the moment, to find the best combination of associations to explain the case. In order to make maximal sense, writes Cavell, the analyst "will have weighed one set of beliefs and desires in the light of others and in the light of his ongoing perceptions of events in the world. Therefore, as [the patient's] interpreter there is in principle no end to the adjustments in interpretation I will be prepared to make. A belief or desire of [the patient's] that I find senseless in the context of one mental structure may reveal its sense in the light of another" (1988, p. 604). The alternatives are weighed in the service of maximizing the coherence of the package; as coherence is increased, understanding is reinforced. The patient, after all, wants to make sense of his associations in a way that takes account of the greatest number of items. To be told that he follows a general law often tends to reduce the patient to a statistic and make him feel less understood.

Coherence and Correspondence Theories

In highlighting the contrast between an explanation that follows some general law and one that takes fullest advantage of the particular features of the situation, we are pointing up the classical distinction between coherence and correspondence theories of truth. Careful inspection of a particular clinical situation would suggest that the good analyst subscribes to a coherence theory. He is more interested in how a particular set of associations fit together (coherence) than in whether they correspond to some general law. But in publishing his observations (as we will see in a later chapter) he is tempted to fall back on the more highly regarded correspondence theory and claim membership in normal science.

One of the criticisms often leveled against the coherence theory of truth is that the mere fact that a story can be told about a set of associations does not by itself guarantee the truth of that story. Coherence too often reduces to plausibility, which has been called "a last-refuge tactic for drawing conclusions [because] plausibility can easily become the refuge of, if not scoundrels, analysts who are too ready to jump to conclusions" (Miles and Huberman, 1984, pp. 216–217; quoted in Packer and Addison, 1989, p. 281). But if many of the associations discovered in the analysis of a particular dream or symptom are specific to the occasion, it follows that they cannot possibly correspond to a general theoretical template. What is more, it would seem that attempts to make them correspond will tempt the clinician to treat apples and oranges as the same and to minimize important distinctions in favor of supporting the received theory.

Not only is the full set of associations specific to a particular patient in a specific time and place, but the conclusions derived from this material and the understanding which is negotiated between patient and analyst are almost certainly not repeatable. They would very likely be different if another analyst were in charge of the case, and they might well be different if they occurred (to the same analyst and patient) at a different time in the treatment. It is always the full context that must be taken into account, and because the contents of the analyst's consciousness will always be in flux, his sense of a particular constellation of associations will necessarily vary from session to session. Even if the contents stayed the same, the parts that were uppermost in his awareness, and therefore most impinging on his evaluation of the clinical material, would almost certainly change from one hour to the next, in the process affecting his sense of the "meaning" of the material and therefore the form and content of his interpretations.

Cavell has argued (following Davidson, 1980), that "it is unlikely that anything in the structure of matter reflects the structure of reasons . . . Now we can begin to see that the causal relations traced by a mental description of events might be quite different from those traced by a description of them as physical . . . I can understand why you deeply resent your mother . . . without being able to cite some general law of which this is an instance" (1988, p. 605). We lack general laws in part because any particular combination of clinical happenings, if pursued far enough, has never occurred before; it is their specific sense of contingency that stands out above all and demands a new and different account (and accounting). But if the combination has never occurred before, it follows that any attempt to invoke the correspondence theory of truth will necessarily falsify the overall picture and force unique happenings into an inappropriate and stereotyped matrix. This kind of forcing seems to happen with inexperienced analysts, who feel weighed down by conventional formulations and who lack the wisdom (and sometimes the imagination) to make up rules as they go; it also seems to happen in "wild" analysis when the therapist fails to listen to the full set of clinical happenings (see Schafer, 1985) and is tempted to make a premature (and overly dogmatic) interpretation.

Searching for correspondence fails for another reason, having to do with the peculiar properties of psychic reality. Many of the objects in the patient's associations are composites of real people and make-believe, imaginary companions. Part of the analyst's task is to deconstruct these composites and help the patient distinguish fact from fantasy. But this deconstruction can never be complete. As a result, the clinical material is always peopled with a set of semi-mythical figures, and the truth of the stories about these figures can never be checked against the outside world. Hence, it seems pointless to rely on a correspondence theory when there is often nothing to check against, nothing for the clinical material to correspond to. It could be argued that thinking in correspondence terms tends to transform therapy into mere history taking because history, by and large, refers to something that has left a verifiable record. Once the clinician accepts the fact that he has entered a world with a minimum of real benchmarks—the world of psychic reality—then he must also realize that coherence is his most reliable guide.

The fact that clinical happenings are always understood in context places a particularly heavy burden on the reporting clinician because the details by themselves are not sufficient. In order to properly communicate the way in which the clinical facts hang together, the reporting clinician must also be able to make public a good portion of his conscious mental life at the moment when the clinical happening occurred. We need to know what he was thinking because it is through these thoughts that the clinical details acquire their specific meaning. If we are deprived of this particular context of consciousness, then we either take the details at their face value, assuming there is one, or assimilate them to the conventional stereotype. Misunderstanding is the inevitable result.

We now begin to see how a reliance on the coherence theory of truth places special demands on the clinical report. We are once again reminded of the guiding assumption of the medieval scientist: the specimen is sacred and needs to be exhaustively explored. Something of this fascination with the moment can be found in Freud's more extended dream analyses, because he tries to situate them in time and place and give us the full context of his inner life at the moment when the dream appeared. As we relive these moments with him, the dream details often take on a more significant meaning. What is more important, their emotional lading becomes more and more transparent, and we find ourselves reacting to the personages in the dream in ways that parallel his reactions. As our awareness of the dream details begins to mimic Freud's, we cannot help but find ourselves understanding his reactions more clearly. The dream is no longer a foreign body—an exotic specimen—but something that we might have dreamt ourselves. Once that step is taken, understanding is significantly enhanced.

But where Freud's dream specimens are the primary examples of this kind of coherence analysis, supplying us with enough context to make even the doubtful details all but transparent, more contemporary samples of clinical reporting tend to be undernourished and leave too much inference up to the reader. As a result, they tend to be unconvincing at best and unreadable at worst. They are no longer clinical specimens in either the botanical or medieval sense of the word. Their faults tend to stem from one of three tendencies. In some cases, the author has unwittingly projected part of the necessary context of understanding onto the reader (also known as the projective fallacy; see Spence, 1982, p. 248); at other times, he has given up his medieval heritage too quickly and taken on the conventions of modern science, attempting to use general laws to explain specific clinical happenings; and finally, he has settled for a pedestrian description of the target event, either casting it in stereotypical language that fails to capture its immediacy or restricting his account to theoretical unobservables that fail to capture its full flavor.

Failures of the third kind bring up the issue of rhetoric once again, and we begin to see that skill in language use is central to providing an account that may be shared. Stein (1988) has written about the importance of providing a coherent and well-organized narrative account when putting a clinical happening into words. Without these features, he argues, the clinical report remains blurred and uncommunicable. It also remains unconvincing. With almost no exceptions, the moment being described is one that never happened before, either to the treating analyst or to his readers. If details are omitted, it tends to be assimilated to moments that have happened and unlikely or improbable conclusions are likely to follow. Moreover, if sufficient details are not provided, the reader will unwittingly project onto the description aspects of clinical happenings he has experienced in his own practice as a way of normalizing the moment and putting it into an understandable frame of reference. He may even achieve a kind of coherence, but the pattern being formed is *his* pattern and has little if any resemblance to the one-of-a-kind pattern originally described by the treating analyst.

We begin to understand more clearly one of the persistent problems in clinical reporting: unique patterns must be described in a way that makes them transparent to someone who has never seen them before. In choosing coherence over correspondence, we have the special problem of describing the unique in a manner that makes it more or less transparent. Yet too often the description is compromised: unlikely clinical happenings are reduced to a set of misleading principles so that some kind of understanding takes place. But the quest for coherence among outside readers tends to destroy the coherence within the clinical happening, and it is the latter that is truly singular and deserves to be protected at all costs. To put the paradox another way, we can argue that the unique clinical happening, if described in a way that is true to the richness of the specimen, will very likely never be completely understood and the treating analyst will find himself a prisoner of his own experience. Thus the need for understanding will probably destroy the specimen.

Awareness of which details to highlight and which to suppress requires one kind of rhetorical skill; an understanding of which details need further explaining requires a second; and the ability to identify with the reader and see and hear the material for the first time requires a third.

Not only does the clinician's reliance on the coherence theory of truth place a heavy burden on the form and content of his narrative account, but it also carries the implication that no explanation is final. This knowledge was also part of the conceptualist medieval heritage and accounted for part of the fascination with the favorite specimen. As new details were uncovered, either in the target object or in the context of discovery, new understandings would follow. Careful study and restudy of cherished specimens was thought to be the expected role of the scholar, whose mission it was to build up a near-complete understanding of the specific object of study and not to enlarge upon the general laws of science—a concept for which, at that time, there was no proper label.

II

The Rhetorical Voice

4 Metaphor as Theory

The presence of the rhetorical voice has been evident almost since the beginning of psychoanalysis, but it is only recently that this mode of discourse has attracted much attention. Some commentators take heart in the discovery of rhetoric because it seems to free psychoanalysis from the traditional constraints of science and give added weight to the "hermeneutic turn." Others have expressed a concern that the rhetorical voice is unnecessarily persuasive, that it carries more influence than seems appropriate, somehow diluting the pure voice of reason. Still others—perhaps the majority—have assumed that although rhetoric has its faults, it is only a temporary expedient, a passing phase that will disappear as soon as better terms are discovered and psychoanalysis is grounded firmly on a secure foundation.

Writing to Jung in 1911, Freud admitted that "I was not at all cut out to be an inductive researcher—I was entirely meant for intuition" (cited in Mahony, 1987, p. 17). "Like a good rhetorician," writes Mahony, Freud "knew that the rhetorical counterpart of inductive proof in scientific demonstration was the example, whose logical frailty demanded the support and distraction of persuasive maneuvers" (p. 168). We have seen that Freud began his scientific career by following traditional inductivist principles and that he turned away from this kind of science at about the time he began to lose faith in his theory of seduction (around the turn of the century). Since that time, the force of psychoanalytic argument has tended to rely more on rhetorical persuasion than on an appeal to data.

Rhetoric has been defined as the "art of using language for persuasion, in speaking or writing" (Cuddon, 1977, p. 557). Vickers (1988) calls it the "art of persuasive communication" long recognized "as the systematization of natural eloquence" (p. 1). It has traditionally relied on a wide range of figures of speech to carry out this task—some authorities cite over two hundred available tropes—but over the years, as rhetoric has declined in popularity and influence, this choice has narrowed down to *metonomy, metaphor,* and *simile* (with one or two others making an occasional appearance).

Part of the decline stems directly from success. Ever since Plato mounted the first attack against it, critics of rhetoric have felt it to be an unfair weapon that must be suppressed at all costs, a suspect art that

> subordinates knowledge to action and reason to will. It aligns persuasion and passion. It takes its place next to the arts, but claims for itself some of the functions of philosophy. It enjoins orators to feel passion, but does not forbid them to feign it. It does not require passion, even if actually felt, to be genuinely justified by the facts. Since orators must be able to argue either side of every issue, their passion need be no more than a state into which they work themselves the better to manipulate their audience . . . Such are the reasons that account for rhetoric's current ill repute. Indifferent to the truth, it is associated with speech or writing elegant in form but empty in content, or with modes of communication which, by means of clever linguistic devices, mislead their audience into unjustified conclusions or decisions. (Nehamas, 1988, p. 771)

The "rhetorical voice" of psychoanalysis can refer, at the most obvious level, to the prevalence of metaphor in Freud's theoretical formulations. This stylistic virtue (or defect, depending on your point of view) was characteristic of Freud's writings from the beginning and seemed to trouble him much less than it did his followers. In *Die Traumdeutung,* he sets forth his position as follows:

> I see no necessity to apologize for the imperfections of this or of any similar imagery. Analogies of this kind are only intended to assist us in our attempt to make the complications of mental functioning intelligible by dissecting the function and assigning its different constituents to different component parts of the apparatus. So far as I know, the experiment has not hitherto been made of using this method of dissection in order to investigate the way in which the mental instrument is put together, and I can see no harm in it. We are justified, in my view, in giving free rein to our speculations so long as we retain the coolness of our judgment and do not mistake the scaffolding for

the building. And since at our first approach to something unknown all that we need is the assistance of provisional ideas, I shall give preference in the first instance to hypotheses of the crudest and most concrete description. (Freud, 1900, p. 536; quoted in Wurmser, 1977, p. 473)

Two points should be noted: the scaffolding should not be mistaken for the building and the use of analogies is particularly useful in the beginning ("in the first instance") as a way of comprehending the unknown. Some years later, in a more formal statement of the same theme, Freud carried the argument a step further. Science always depends, he wrote, on nebulous concepts "which it hopes to apprehend more clearly in the course of its development, or which it is even prepared to replace by others" (1914, p. 77). Thus metaphor, while initially useful, should be seen as a temporary expedient that will be abandoned when the referent in question comes more clearly into focus.

The rhetorical voice does not confine itself to the reliance on metaphor (and other standard tropes) in psychoanalytic language; it also speaks in other ways that have received less explicit attention. The recent focus on the narrative aspects of the psychoanalytic discourse (see Schafer, 1976; Spence, 1982) also raises rhetorical questions in a context that goes beyond the use of specific figures of speech. If the form of an interpretation (for example, its "narrative fit"; see Spence, 1982) plays a role in its effect on the patient, then questions of rhetoric bear directly on questions of technique. If narrative truth should be distinguished from historical truth, then rhetorical issues begin to take on more importance in the way we listen to patients and in the way we frame interpretations.

The role of rhetoric also comes into play in the way we study Freud. If the specific content of the Irma dream and its associations affect the way we are persuaded by Freud's argument about the role of infantile wishes, then the influence of his theory rests partly on rhetorical issues that need to be examined. Similar questions apply to the case histories. It goes without saying that a reading of the Dora case has a significantly greater impact on the beginning analyst than a mere listing of its major points; this greater impact is one reason why it is required reading in almost all institutes, and why the *Standard Edition* still serves as our primary text. Thus it would seem that it is partly for rhetorical reasons that we are still very much in Freud's shadow.

Last of all, we come to the good and bad features of the case study genre. The five case histories are perhaps the clearest examples of Freud's rhetorical voice, and the case history tradition under which we still work tends to place a heavy emphasis on narrative and literary considerations. "To convey the sense and atmosphere of an analytic experience," writes Stein, "means that we must tell a coherent story about it, a truthful one, but a story nevertheless. The preparation of a good clinical report requires a reorganization and selection of data without which the material remains inchoate and incapable of being communicated in a useful fashion" (1988, p. 114). Just how to perform this feat is still a matter of debate, but it seems clear that the nature of the story and the conviction it conveys depend on issues of narrative and rhetorical persuasion. Effective clinical writing, as Freud was the first to recognize, shares many of the virtues of good fiction, and much depends on how the material is selected and presented. The importance of rhetoric thus comes clearly into focus.

The Role of Metaphor

In one of his earliest statements on the matter, Freud pointed to the importance of beginning with tentative, indefinite ideas that have been imposed on the clinical observations. These initial formulations "are in the nature of conventions—although everything depends on their not being arbitrarily chosen but determined by their having significant relations to the empirical material, relations that we seem to sense before we can clearly recognize and demonstrate them. It is only after more thorough investigation of the field of observation that we are able to formulate its basic scientific concepts with increased precision, and progressively so to modify them that they become serviceable and consistent over a wide area" (1915, p. 117). These ideas can be readily replaced because they "are not the foundation of science, upon which everything rests; that foundation is observation alone. They are not the bottom but the top of the whole structure, and they can be replaced and discarded without damaging it" (1914, p. 77).

The idea of replacement soon became the point at issue. Thus Hartmann notes that "an occasional lack of caution in the formulation of its propositions, or Freud's liking for occasional striking metaphors, has led to the accusation against analysis of an anthropomorphization of its concepts. But *in all these cases* a more careful formulation can be substituted which will dispell this impression" (1959; quoted in Grossman and Simon, 1969, p. 79; italics mine).

If the metaphor was not replaced, damage could result, and Hartmann, Kris, and Loewenstein (1946) spell out the two sides of the question:

> Clearly, whenever dramatization is encountered, metaphorical language has crept into scientific discourse and that there is danger in the use of metaphor hardly needs to be demonstrated . . . However, it remains a problem worth some further discussion, under what conditions the danger outweighs the advantage. The danger obviously begins if and when metaphor infringes upon meaning; in the case in point, when structural concepts are anthropomorphized. Then the functional connotations may be lost and one of the psychic systems may be substituted for the total personality. (Quoted in Grossman and Simon, 1969, p. 81)

Nagel (1959) provided one way in which metaphor could infringe on meaning. "In Freudian theory," he wrote, "metaphors are employed without even halfway definite rules for expanding them and . . . in consequence, admitted metaphors such as 'energy' or 'level of excitation' have no specific content and can be filled to suit one's fancy" (quoted in Wurmser, 1977, p. 476). Other critics of metaphor, while generally not as disapproving as Nagel, have tended to agree with Freud that it is at best a temporary expedient and will one day be replaced when the phenomena are seen more clearly or when the theory has become more sophisticated.

Up until about 1969, the rhetorical voice of psychoanalysis was never very loud and was treated as an embarrassing intruder, clearly inferior to the evidential voice that would command general attention when metaphors were replaced by the appropriate technical language. But with the publication in 1969 of Grossman and Simon's landmark paper on the virtues of anthropomorphic usage, with particular respect to the clinical theory, the rhetorical voice began to command more respect. Grossman and Simon argued, first, that introspective experience is naturally described in anthropomorphic terms, and thus in their early stages, psychoanalytic concepts will quite naturally be rendered in similar images. It follows that from the clinical theory, "it is not necessary to 'purge' anthropomorphic language. Anthropomorphic language is in no way incompatible with systematic study of individual cases" and in many applications—for example, when referring to such processes as wishing, intending, and needing—"there is no other language available" (p. 108). Schafer's (1976) work on action language—an attempt to get rid of metaphor—had yet to appear.

Grossman and Simon also took a more careful look at the question of metaphor replacement and showed why attempts to use hydraulic or electrical models to explain the workings of the mind are generally unsatisfactory. They fail, first, because they are physical conceptualizations and therefore lack empathy, lending an "impersonal quality to the formulation." Second, the abstract tidiness of the formulation is frequently misleading because its essential function cannot be mathematically expressed and its terms cannot be interrelated and connected into some larger, overarching theory. Third, the model has no "referent other than the observation metaphorically represented" (p. 100). I will return to the problem of the vanishing referent in a later section.

Turning to the higher-level theory, Grossman and Simon seemed of two minds. Although they regarded metaphor as a beginning explanation pointing toward a more comprehensive theory, as I have noted, they were dissatisfied with attempts to substitute one image for another. Thus, they seemed to argue that metaphor should be replaced, but they were much less optimistic than Hartmann that the chances of finding a suitable substitute were good, nor did they suggest exactly where the improvements would come from.

More recently, the rhetorical voice has been given enthusiastic support by Wurmser (1977), Wallerstein (1988), and Spence (1987). Wurmser came to the explicit defense of metaphor in theory formation and argued not only that metaphors are indispensable but that we need more of them (p. 494). "All science," he wrote, "is the systematic use of metaphor" (p. 477). In his 1987 presidential address to the International Psychoanalytic Association, Wallerstein repeats and expands on Wurmser's appeal and continues the distinction between clinical theory and metapsychology developed by Grossman and Simon. In agreement with them, he takes the position that, with respect to clinical theory, metaphor creates no problem because clinical facts are "sufficiently experience-near, anchored directly enough to observables, to the data of our consulting room, that [theory] is amenable to the self-same processes of hypothesis formation, testing, and validation as any other scientific enterprise" (1988, p. 17). With respect to metatheory, Wallerstein takes a more pessimistic position on replacement and a stronger position on metaphor. In place of the conclusion that metaphor functions as a temporary expedient, someday to be replaced by something more descriptively apt, Wallerstein reads the "different and distinguishing theoretical positions . . . that mark our psychoanalytic pluralism . . . as primarily metaphors" that are "beyond the realm of empirical study and scientific process" (p. 17). In other words, our larger theory does not rest on metaphor as a temporary expedient; it *is* largely metaphor and will probably remain that way. The rhetorical voice is in full cry.

I have also argued (1987, Chap. 1) that our current theory is largely metaphorical and should thus be seen as a collection of hypotheses, tentative models of the workings of the mind that are still in their early phases of development, and should not be prematurely frozen into established theory. I also point out that the choice of any one metaphor or model always implies the discarding of another. If we lock ourselves into the more familiar metaphors too quickly, we lose the possibility of arriving at other models that may better mesh with the clinical findings. Because the stuff of the mind is largely out of reach, it is particularly important that we respect the distinction between metaphor and referent by keeping the metaphor alive. Once it becomes a simple matter of description (a "dead" metaphor), we have been fooled by language into thinking that we know more than we do.

> To keep the Freudian approach alive as metaphor is to extract its fullest potential and to make the greatest use of other options when the need requires. To speak metaphorically in full awareness of this fact is to be reminded that we are using language figuratively and tentatively—but at the same time, extending its use in significant ways. But to take the Freudian system for granted—to deaden the metaphor and rule out other approaches—is to reduce our options to only one and mistakenly transform metaphor into pseudo-science. To use it in this way is to diminish the poetry of Freud's original inspiration and, in the long run, to miss the spirit of the whole adventure. (Spence, 1987, p. 8)

Can Metaphor Be Replaced?

Freud had hoped that extended clinical observations would sharpen the earlier, tentative formulations, make them more precise, and eventually prepare them for inclusion in an overarching theory. Similar hopes were shared by Hartmann, Grossman and Simon, and many other commentators, and, with respect to the clinical theory, by Wallerstein. But psychoanalytic observations are not only theory-laden and mediated by implicit models, they are also constrained by the fact that many of our central terms—such as the unconscious—are, by definition, not observable. It is probably no accident that the language used to describe this concept has not changed substantially over the last one hundred years, and while we may no longer really believe that it is a "cauldron full of seething excitations" or that repressed, instinctual representatives "proliferate in the dark," we are hard-pressed to make direct contact with the referent and improve on our description.

The philosopher Richard Boyd has drawn detailed attention to the crucial role played by metaphor in the development of any scientific theory. What he calls "theory-constitutive metaphors" are used for "expressing theoretical claims for which no adequate literal paraphrase is known" (1979, p. 360). Boyd uses the term "epistemic access" to describe the link between metaphor and referent; the well-chosen metaphor allows us to refine our method of observation so that we see the phenomenon more clearly, which, in turn, leads to modifications in the terms of explanation. It is this feedback, "this sort of linguistically-mediated epistemic success—*which necessarily includes modification of linguistic usage to accommodate language to newly discovered causal features of the world*—[which] is the very core of reference" (pp. 398–399; italics in the original).

But it is difficult to see how this approach can be applied to many of our favorite and most useful concepts. Even though the unconscious is "experience-near" (to use Wallerstein's phrase), it is neither open to introspection (by definition) nor to any kind of description, linguistic or otherwise; thus no metaphor, no matter how artfully chosen, can provide true epistemic access. And because the unconscious is so shielded, no metaphor used to describe it can ever be fully disallowed.

It is here that we are most vulnerable to the rhetorical voice of psychoanalysis. Metaphors that are used to describe clinical happenings not open to direct observation can never, it would seem, be further refined by more extended observation; as a result, they may never be replaced. But because it is hard to believe that we must ground our theory and our practice on purely figurative language, we are tempted to overlook the metaphorical essence of the former and treat it as standard wisdom. In this way, what is really metaphor turns into accepted knowledge—the rhetorical voice has bested the evidential voice—but remains unrecognized because of our bias against "mere rhetoric."

We can detect an antirhetorical bias in any argument to get rid of metaphor (or any other trope) and replace it with a "more careful formulation." The graphic figures of speech used by Freud are not merely too approximate and imprecise, they are also stained by their membership in the family of standard rhetorical tropes that are "clever devices" designed to "mislead their audience." While Mahony's (1987) masterful summary of Freud's style can be read on a purely descriptive level, one can also sense the implicit warning that the reader should watch out for such figures as enargia (the pictorial rendering of a scene, which we encountered in Chapter 2) and *chiasmus* (the repetition of words in reverse order) lest he be caught off guard and find himself persuaded against his will. Only when all doubtful terms have been replaced will we be secure against the rhetorical voice. It can be seen that in this view, the rhetorical voice is one of irrationality at the other extreme from the evidential voice of pure reason.

Where Are the Facts?

In his initial essay on the problem in *Die Traumdeutung*, Freud cautioned against mistaking the scaffolding for the building. Perhaps it is just this confusion that identifies our current predicament. Lacking direct access to the stuff of the mind, we are quick to substitute convenient metaphors; because they can never be checked, they are prone to shift, gradually and silently, from hypothesis to explanation and, in the process, to obscure the fact that, in reality, almost nothing is known for certain. Skinner has recently drawn attention to the fact that very little agreement exists about the principal achievements of psychology, and he notes that when ten psychologists were asked to name the most important discoveries made during a fifteen-year period, no two of them could agree (1987, p. 784). Similar disagreements might be expected with regard to psychoanalysis. Not only have we failed to build a *cumulative* set of findings over the past one hundred years, but because we cannot make contact with the stuff of the mind, we have no way of knowing the actual relationship that may exist between different hypothetical systems. This problem is rooted in our fondness for figurative language. While many of our favorite expressions are vivid and almost poetic in their specificity (clear examples, it would seem, of enargia), each expression is entirely self-contained; each trope draws on a specific frame of reference and gives us no information about its relation to other descriptive terms. Thus, we may feel comfortable, even intrigued, by the comparison of the psychic apparatus with a telescope and find ourselves fascinated by Freud's argument that all objects of internal perception can be thought of as "virtual, like the image produced in a telescope by the passage of light-rays. And . . . we may compare the censorship between two systems to the refraction which takes place when a ray of light passes into a new medium" (1900, p. 611). But this metaphor tells us nothing about the "space" in which this action takes place. If we feel "filled with anger," does this refer to the same space we use in forming the virtual image? We may reply that these expressions are only metaphors, but by what criteria do we know which ones are merely heuristic and which are something more? It was this problem that caused Nagel to point out that psychoanalysis has no "even halfway definite rules" for bridging metaphor and observation.

When considered closely, such terms as "seething cauldron" or "virtual image" or "unconscious fantasy" simply fail to give us epistemic access to the stuff of the mind; they fail to tell us where to look, what to look for, and how to recognize what we've found. They are merely metaphors that masquerade as, and substitute for, explanations. A current, social constructionist view even takes the position that the traditional attempt to establish knowledge of the mind through empirical verification is entirely mistaken. By this argument, there is no mind-stuff to be found, just as there are no facts in the world "out there" to be discovered. "The mind," writes Gergen, "becomes a form of social myth; the self-concept is removed from the head and placed within the sphere of social discourse. In each case . . . what have been taken by one segment of the profession or another as 'facts about the nature of the psychological realm' are suspended; each concept (emotion, motivation, etc.) is cut away from an ontological base within the head and is made a constituent of social process" (1985, p. 271). Not only is Gergen suspicious about the "truth" of mental life; he would probably argue that the failure of psychoanalysis to cash its metaphors only proves that it is seeking to map something that does not exist.

This argument would suggest that psychoanalysis all along has been the victim of language; that what is called clinical intuition or empathy (to take only one example) has fooled us into thinking that the way we talk about feelings or ideas or motivation has some objective referent, whereas, in fact, there may be nothing there. We mistake appearance for reality. Clinical experience, along with a highly figurative theoretical language, has fooled us into thinking that there is mind-stuff inside the head when in fact we are dealing only with words. Thus, we should not be surprised by the fact that either our metaphors are always changing or, if established, they never seem to make contact with the "facts."

We are also the victims of a scientific century. To speak about the *laws* of primary and secondary process, for example, is to further the possibility that the mind is merely another object of study and that the stuff of the mind is organized according to standard rules that remain to be discovered. This line of thinking not only reflects our technological bias, as Sampson (1981) has shown, it also protects us from what Bernstein (1983) has called the Cartesian anxiety—the fear that nothing is fixed and that, in the last analysis, nothing is known: "Either there is some support for our being, a fixed foundation for our knowledge, or we cannot escape the forces of darkness that envelop us with madness, with intellectual and moral chaos . . . At the heart of the objectivist's vision, and what makes sense of his or her passion, is the belief that there are or must be some fixed, permanent constraints to which we can appeal and which are secure and stable" (pp. 18–19).

Searching for the Evidential Voice

When Freud was first beginning his work, he had high hopes for his "method of dissection," which would make intelligible the functioning of the "mental instrument." As we come to realize that the important stuff of the mind may always be just out of reach, we must make a clear distinction between what Freud hoped to establish (an empiricist science) and what the field has actually become. It would seem that much of the metaphor that is embedded in standard theory will never be replaced; thus it is all the more important that we recognize it for what it is. In taking this step, we give full marks to the rhetorical voice, calling it by its proper name.

Where is the evidential voice? It is only gradually making itself heard, and in the last chapter we will have a chance to listen to it more carefully. But because most of the metaphors will probably never be replaced (and because psychoanalysis is not truly a Galilean science) it seems unlikely that our favorite figures of speech will give way to the "more careful formulation" that Hartmann thought was always available. The rhetorical voice, in other words, may be our primary source of information about the clinical happening for some time to come. Made uncomfortable by the "softness" of Freud's rhetorical voice and impressed by its promise of better things to come (including the hope of membership in normal science), we are tempted to sit back and wait for the scaffolding to be removed and the building to appear. But we are now beginning to realize that the building we are seeking may have quite a different shape and location, that it is not even concealed by the scaffolding. Perhaps scaffolding and building are in fact one and the same.

I am purposely using one of Freud's rhetorical figures to illustrate our dependence on the rhetorical tradition. It is hard to see how the point could be made in any other fashion. Shortly after writing this comment, I came across the following apology from Freud, which makes the same point: In "being obliged to operate with the figurative language peculiar to psychology, we could not otherwise describe the processes in question at all, and indeed we could not have become aware of them" (1920, p. 60).

Where, once again, is the evidential voice of psychoanalysis? When it appears, can it be trusted? If he is too eager to join the ranks of hard science, the clinician tends to water down the clinical happening and express it in terms of standard (often dead) metaphors, inadequate necessary truths and partial covering laws, making us believe that the received theory has been confirmed. But in the process, the unique clarity of the observation is usually lost and so is the matter being described. Occasional glimpses of unexpected phenomena have appeared in the literature from time to time, but they tend to be co-opted by the conventional metaphors, which make us believe that standard theory has been confirmed. Every time a piece of new evidence has been captured in this way, we have probably lost the chance to make an important new discovery. It is partly for this reason that psychoanalysis lacks the cumulative thrust of the other sciences.

Borrowing Paul Valéry's comment on history, we could say from one point of view that psychoanalysis "is the most dangerous product evolved from the chemistry of the intellect . . . [It] will justify anything.

It teaches precisely nothing, for it contains everything and furnishes examples of everything" (quoted in White, 1978, p. 36). It is precisely because the theory ranges so widely that the voice of empty rhetoric—the reductive voice—is so hard to shut out. It has a place for everything. It is hard to think of a single clinical observation that would not find a home in the standard theory.

But finding a home—finding a name for the clinical discovery—is not the same as finding an explanation. For that task, we need to develop ever more precise descriptions of selected clinical specimens. In the process, we may achieve the proper level of what Geertz has called "thick description." Such description would capture the clinical gist of a happening in a way that would satisfy all commentators. Once we arrive at that point, we could begin to develop a technical language to describe the happening in a way that goes beyond metaphor. When we take that step, we have fulfilled Hartmann's hope for a more careful formulation. We are able, at long last, to "formulate [our] basic scientific concepts with increased precision, and progressively so to modify them that they become serviceable and consistent over a wide area" (Freud, 1915, p. 117). In Chapter 9, we will begin to move in this direction by replacing the metaphor of analytic surface with concepts that are more easily objectified. I would hope that similar replacements can be accomplished in other areas. As our powers of "thick description" grow stronger, we can learn to become more suspicious of empty rhetoric and find ways to immunize ourselves against its more reductive attempts. And as clinical specimens begin to accumulate, we will finally have the data base we need to sharpen our favorite concepts and enrich our descriptions.

Does this line of argument mean that psychoanalysis will eventually give up its rhetorical voice? It is the hope of perhaps the majority of psychoanalysts that metaphor will someday be replaced by more precise language and that when that day comes, we can unashamedly join the ranks of twentieth-century science. But this hope discounts the extent to which psychoanalysis is grounded in the Aristotelian tradition, a tradition that supports metaphor (and other rhetorical figures) as a perfectly justified mode of description and explanation. If our discipline is truly conceptualist in its orientation, then any attempt to make its formulations more abstract, quantitative, and general may bring about a paradoxical decrease in precision. In trying too precipitously to ape the hard sciences, we will necessarily abandon our birthright. On the other hand, a full awareness of the rhetorical and conceptualist foundation of our discipline should make us more observant clinicians, who are concerned about providing full (and persuasive) descriptions wherever possible. In assuming this role, we learn to "surrender" ourselves to the clinical happening and its contingent truth. Once that task is accomplished, we are in a position to explore the full richness of a specimen that has never happened before and will never happen again (in quite that way), and which thus demands the utmost in our choice of language to make it come alive for the reader.

This line of argument returns us to the importance of the specimen—both in the Aristotelian tradition and in current clinical practice. If we take its importance seriously, we need to begin to build a public data base that captures significant clinical happenings and preserves them in a way that does not violate their original meaning. The American Psychoanalytic Association has published a set of guidelines for case presentations (see Klumpner and Frank, 1991). These guidelines propose that every published case should contain a short, near-verbatim interchange between analyst and patient. They make detailed distinctions between verbatim quotation and paraphrase, and between what was spoken and what was thought. They also propose formats for including original dialogue and commentaries on this dialogue, written either by the treating analyst or by an outside observer.

As these clinical excerpts begin to accumulate, we have the start of a clinical archive. In *The Freudian Metaphor* (Spence, 1987), I have argued that detailed specimens are important because the clinical wisdom lies in the detail. The same argument was an important part of the conceptualist tradition. But where the medieval scientist felt that only the gifted observer was in a position to understand the complexity of the specimen fully, I am making the argument that a suitably presented specimen will be perfectly clear to *any* reader. To make this possible—to understand the meaning of an utterance at the time it was uttered—it seems necessary to illuminate the clinical happening through the commentary of the treating analyst and a range of commentaries from significant others, patients included. Robert Stoller has appealed to the need to include more of the patient's point of view. He urges us to "develop a new rhetoric in which our patients' positions are visible. Doing so may also help us to develop more rigorous, as well as more readable, less jargon-soaked argument" (1988, p. 385).

Testimony from patients, as we all realize, is conspicuous by its absence. As we begin to listen to and learn from this voice, we may begin to make our most exciting discoveries.

As clinical data begin to accumulate, certain specimens, either because they illuminate a particular clinical issue or offer a good example of a standard theoretical concept, might take on the standing of landmark cases in the law (see Spence, 1987, Chap. 6). As these specimens are identified, they would begin to provide the referents for specific theoretical concepts. Thus a particular kind of transference might be linked to a particular clinical happening and in this way, theoretical terms would become grounded in specific detail. I would note the emphasis on specificity. We are not searching for a covering law (necessary truth) that would define all examples of transference in the way a law of gravity describes all falling objects. We are still grounded in the particular and remain faithful to the complexity of the specimen. But whereas the medieval scientist would probably make the better specimens part of a secret order, we are trying to bring them into the public domain.

With specimen happenings as reference points for critical parts of the theory, the way is clear to find the best set of terms and the best combination of words that will capture the gist of the clinical event and preserve it forever. Benchmark specimens will constrain our use of mere metaphor and stand in the way of a frivolous use of language. And while our metaphors may never provide epistemic access to the stuff of the mind, they can and do point to specific clinical encounters. We expect that the meaning of these encounters will gradually change as a result of peer discussion; as the meaning changes, the rhetorical presentations will also evolve. In this way, theory follows closely on observation, and language lives up to its full potential.

The Dangers of Empty Rhetoric

The program I have just outlined is, unfortunately, more easily described than carried out, largely because the rhetorical voice of psychoanalysis has lulled us into believing that we understand far more than we actually do. We are also tempted to believe that any direct challenge to the master's authority is in bad taste and betrays an unseemly lack of respect for good science and clinical sensitivity. The rhetorical voice of Freud's five cases persuades us that the essential clinical questions presented by his patients have already been answered by standard theory. If we read these cases enough times, we lose our sense of what is not explained and end up giving way to Freud's masterful narrative voice, whose effect grows stronger on each new hearing. This is one of the reasons why the five cases play such an important role in the standard psychoanalytic curriculum.

But as the newer deconstructionist critics are beginning to make clear, the classic cases rest on debatable logic and inconclusive evidence, and once their rhetoric is stripped away, their persuasive impact is significantly diminished. One of the more telling critiques is Stanley Fish's (1986) analysis of the Wolf Man case. He devotes particular attention to the extent to which the clinical insights from the case were stage-managed by Freud rather than being the spontaneous products of the patient's free associations. In such sentences as "It required a long education to persuade and induce [the patient] to take an independent share of the work," we begin to gain an understanding of the artful way in which Freud both masterminded the story and concealed his role in its production.

"Always," writes Fish, "the pattern is the same: the claims of independence—for the analysis, for the patient's share, for the 'materials'—is made in the context of an account that powerfully subverts it, and then it is made again" (p. 935). While on the one hand we begin to sense the power of Freud's influence on the emerging material, on the other our suspicions are continually disabled by Freud's assertion that suggestion is out of the question. At one point he tells us that "it is unjust [sic] to attribute the results of analysis to the physician's imagination," at another, that he finds it "impossible even to argue with those who regard the findings of psychoanalysis as 'artifacts.'" "These and similar statements," Fish says, "would seem to suggest that his motives are not personal, but institutional; he speaks not for himself but on behalf of the integrity of a discipline." But the discipline

is one of which he is quite literally the father, and his defense of its integrity involves him in the same contradiction that marks his relationship with the patient and the reader: no sooner has he insisted on the independence of psychoanalysis as a science than he feels compelled to specify, and to specify authoritatively, what the nature of that science is; and once he does that he is in the untenable position of insisting on the autonomy of something of which he is unable to let go. (1986, p. 935)

Fish helps us see that by repeatedly denying the charge of suggestion, by pretending to dismiss it on almost moral grounds, by making the point that he is presenting us only with the facts—and supported by Strachey's announcement (in the preface of Freud's *Introductory Lectures*) that Freud was "never rhetorical"—Freud manages to persuade all but the most convinced skeptic that his story is a true account of the clinical happenings of the Wolf Man case. By implication he tells us that any sign of doubt would be not only disloyal but evidence of agreeing with the enemy (Jung and Adler). We are no longer in a position to choose freely among alternatives, much less in a position to look at all the data and construct our own version; we must decide whether we are with him or against him. Questions of evidence and interpretation become questions of loyalty, and the hopeful reader— or still worse, the anxious candidate—has no choice but to accept the verdict of the master.

Fish makes it possible for us to see the rhetorical depth of the Wolf Man case, and under his guidance we begin to read it with somewhat clearer eyes. But this is a difficult task because we are haunted, from the outset, by thoughts that we are being disloyal to Freud and the psychoanalytic tradition, and we find ourselves with the worrying thought that Fish is only a mischief-maker, up to no good, and therefore someone to be ignored.

Thoughts of this kind speak to the difficulty we face in setting aside the rhetorical voice of psychoanalysis and dealing only with the facts. Despite Strachey's disclaimer, rhetoric has been part of its appeal from the beginning, and one of its hidden themes has been the doubtful standing of the independent thinker. In contrast to the traditions of normal science, there is no precedent in psychoanalysis for the disinterested independent critic who wants to see with his own eyes and develop from these observations his own ideas. From the very beginning, this stance has been implicitly challenged as a sign of bad faith and evidence for unreliability.

Not only has the official rhetoric discouraged independent thought, it has also discouraged any attempt to look long and hard at our metaphoric heritage and recognize its implications. If language is all we have (primarily because many of the referents that matter are essentially out of reach) then we have to be more than usually on guard against the perils of empty rhetoric and authoritarian argument. These were the dangers that Plato had in mind when he warned his pupils against the seductions of elegant writing. We are exposed to these dangers (as we will see more clearly in a later chapter) when confronted with case reports that honor conclusions over evidence, that take Freud's statements as literally true and needing only reconfirmation, that rely too heavily on argument by authority to persuade the reader, that assume that the facts are essentially transparent and thus that the author's interpretation is usually correct, and that rush too quickly from the single incident to the covering law. It could be argued that since meanings in clinical material are *not* transparent, it is all the more necessary that we not fall back on authoritarian forms of argument. To depend on a single opinion (the author/analyst's) is perilous enough; to depend on it when meanings are frequently ambiguous and context-determined is to confound the problem all the more.

It could be argued that our most widely cited case studies are almost never simple reports of clinical happenings but are instead complicated exercises of persuasion that implicitly support established theory. As Stoller comments, "Pick up any issue of a psychoanalytic journal . . . and read at random a clinical description. The report is so much the analyst's version and the writing style applied to the clinical story so free of uncertainty, whether the writer's version of the story is the right one or not, that we automatically accept the description as reality. [On reading the account] you will sense, beyond the innumerable declarative statements that produce a sense of factuality, an ambience—a rhetoric—in which the author's position is the fixed point in the universe, serving as baseline truth" (1988, pp. 384–385).

The dangers of empty rhetoric can be seen more clearly if we turn to Paul Ricoeur's dichotomy (see Ricoeur, 1970, pp. 28–29) and distinguish between an account that reduces the episode to a causal explanation—such as "the patient acted out of sadistic impulses"— and an account that, in Ricoeur's and Gadamer's language, "surrenders" to the particularity of the event and conveys its richness in all the detail necessary to persuade the reader. The first kind of explanation tends to be brief, final, authoritarian, and unconvincing, but it places few demands on the reader. The second calls on the writer to exercise all of his rhetorical skills, exploring not only the clinical happening but his unfolding reaction to it as he gives way to the flow of the material and comes up with an interpretation. For this kind of account, we need to be a participant-observer of the happening in the fullest sense of both roles, now inside the analyst's head as he encounters the material, now standing back and watching the dialogue as it unfolds. It should be clear that capturing this kind of interchange demands rare rhetorical gifts and allows the reader to join the conversation in a way that the first account does not.

But there is still worse to come. Where it was once thought that all useful metaphors could be replaced by consensually validated observations, it now becomes apparent, as we have noted, that metaphor will be with us for a long time. But metaphor alone does not make good science, and as we begin to dismantle the sweeping statements that make up a large part of our theory, the end result will inevitably have much less narrative appeal. Where Freud could say, speaking of his reconstructions of early childhood memories, that "[I] restored what is missing . . . [and] like a conscientious archeologist . . . have not omitted to mention in each case where the authentic parts end and my constructions begin" (1905, p. 12), we would now be forced to say that we often have no way of making this distinction. Where Freud could say that for the analyst "all of the essentials are preserved; even things that seem completely forgotten are present somehow and somewhere" (1937, p. 260), we would have to say that this assertion is largely rhetorical, bears very little relation to the clinical facts, and does not belong in any reliable account. We would have to say that many events seem to be completely forgotten, that the comparison of the mind with an archeological dig is misleading and overly rhetorical, and that there is, at bottom, no evidence that in the unconscious, nothing is forgotten.

Faced with a choice between standard theory on the one hand, with its lofty and irresistible claims, its unsurpassed narrative voice, and its hundred-year history, and the alternative, a stuttering attempt to present an overview of consensually validated clinical findings that depend on only a handful of cases, who would not choose the former? Who would, of his own free will, give up the rolling sentences of the *Standard Edition* and replace them with fragmentary and possibly unreliable accounts of actual clinical happenings written by earnest scientists with no narrative voice and a greater faith in numbers than in words? Would anyone in his right mind want to rewrite Shakespeare?

From one point of view, Freud's extraordinary mixture of insight, observation, and rhetorical flourish can be more easily described as a far-reaching narrative that depends heavily on metaphor and other rhetorical figures to tell a spellbinding tale about the life of the mind than as a testable set of propositions. If we accept the fact that his theory is cast in a narrative mode, then we can take pleasure in reading about the "seething cauldron" of the unconscious, the Censor at the gates of consciousness, and all the other baroque and romantic details in what is called the "Standard Edition." But a clear understanding of its narrative and rhetorical roots should probably prepare us for the likelihood that it will not be translated into pure theory.

Mahony (1987) has made clear many of the rhetorical roots of Freud's style and how much it differs from a series of simple declarative statements. Mistakes will accrue, he writes, if Freud is read for content alone: "The erroneous linking of Freud's prose with the expository discourse of a positive science is reflected in the very nonprocessive, nonprobative style of the commentators who fill English-language psychoanalytic journals" (p. 125). To read him in the narrative mode, on the other hand, is to be open to the particular delights of his style and to realize that much of his writing is taken up with his reflection on what is being presented—the definition of a processive style. Mahony has identified this special feature as belonging to the baroque style of *pensée pensante* (thought thinking). "The reader," he writes, "experiences [in Freud] the ebb and flow of utterances whose harmonization is not present but grasped progressively in cumulatively adjusting perspectives . . . Freud surrendered himself not only to impulse but also to the demands of the material he worked on" (p. 121). As a result, his writing is by turns didactic, rhetorical, serious, playful, straightforward and contradictory—the mark of any good narrative—and, as Mahony makes clear, "the distinctiveness of Freud's presentation is that his talk about the message is at the very heart of the message itself" (p. 136).

What is still missing is a model of clinical reporting that manages to blend rhetorical persuasion with an attention to detail that serves both the best interests of the individual case and the more general theory. I will come back to this question in Chapter 9.

5 Self-Analysis as Justification

A good example of the way in which rhetoric can masquerade as evidence can be found in the legend of Freud's self-analysis. This remarkable story was barely hinted at in *Die Traumdeutung* and only became a central object of study after the publication of the Fleiss letters (Masson, 1985). Since that time, it has attracted the attention of each of Freud's major biographers, and their different versions provide us with multiple examples of how a small number of facts can be rhetorically rearranged to become an enduring legend.

But the legend is much more than that. It can also be read as one of the principal exhibits in the psychoanalytic collection of specimens, one which ranks with the Irma dream and the Dora case as a time-tested distillation of psychoanalytic wisdom. As a classic specimen, it is an object of study that will never yield all its secrets and continues to call for reanalysis and re-inspection. I will first review the rhetorical features of the self-analysis legend, then turn to an examination of the role it plays in grounding the theory in the conceptualist tradition, and finally, examine its role as principal specimen, an obvious object for further study.

Rhetorical Features

We have seen in earlier chapters how both the wealth of detail in *Die Traumdeutung* and the metaphor of discoverer as explorer engaged in mapping out a new country combine to support Freud's credibility as a trustworthy witness. They add significantly to his authority and allow him to present rather extreme conclusions more or less shorn of supporting arguments. We now realize that he is further protected by the daring nature of his expedition. He was not only reporting on dreams, a rather pedestrian subject to which countless others had paid attention, but was also using his dreams to open windows on his past: "I soon saw the necessity of carrying out a self-analysis, and this I did with the help of a series of my own dreams which led me back through all the events of my childhood" (*On the History of the Psychoanalytic Movement*, p. 20; quoted in Clark, 1980, p. 165). The common dream was transformed into a kind of time machine that allowed him to travel into the past; even more remarkably, he seemed able to travel almost at will. In his letter to Fleiss of October 31, 1897, he writes that "everything is still obscure, even the problems, but there is a comfortable feeling in that one has only to reach into one's storerooms to take out what is needed at a particular time" (Masson, 1985, p. 276). "The deeper one carried the analysis of a dream," he tells us in *Die Traumdeutung,* "the more often one comes upon the track of experiences in childhood which have played a part among the sources of that dream's latent content" (1900, p. 198).

The foundation for this kind of time travel lay in Freud's theory of dreams and, in particular, in his view of the role of infantile wishes. Freud was making the revolutionary claim that a wish which is represented in a dream *must* be an infantile wish. "I am aware," he wrote, "that this assertion cannot be proved to hold universally; but it can be proved to hold frequently, even in unsuspected cases, and it cannot be *contradicted* as a general proposition" (1900, pp. 553–554; italics in the original). We see once again Freud's penchant for going from the particular to the general: the assertion is no longer a provisional hypothesis, it has been transformed into an axiom. Liberal use of this proposition enabled him to treat his dreams as derivatives of significant past events ("to our surprise, *we find the child and the child's impulses still living on in the dream*"; 1900, p. 191; italics in the original) and to use associations to these dreams as a means of discovering and reconstructing pieces of his past.

Where is the evidence for this central proposition? What facts support the concept of the wondrous time machine?

> It is true [Freud admitted] that as a rule the childhood scene is only represented in the dream's manifest content by an allusion, and has to be arrived at by an interpretation of the dream. Such instances, when they are recorded, cannot carry much conviction, since as a rule there is no other evidence of these childhood experiences having

occurred; if they date back to a very early age, they are no longer recognized as memories. The general justification for inferring the occurrence of these childhood experiences from dreams is provided by a *whole number of factors in psychoanalytic work* which are mutually consistent and thus seem sufficiently trustworthy. If I record some of these inferred childhood experiences torn from their context for the purposes of dream-interpretation, they may perhaps create little impression, especially as I shall not even be able to quote all the material on which the interpretations were based. Nevertheless I shall not allow this to deter me from relating them. (1900, p. 199; italics mine)

As with so many of Freud's central propositions, the argument is more asserted than derived; we are asked to believe in his conclusions but are not allowed to follow the steps of the argument. The facts presented are, admittedly, not convincing because they are "torn from their context," but if, he seems to imply, we were provided with the full range of psychoanalytic discoveries, we would agree with his conclusions. Notice that by leaving out part of the evidence, Freud adds to our dependence on his authority and, ultimately, on his wisdom. And by referring to unspecified pieces of evidence the reader must take on faith, Freud tends to increase the mystery of his clinical work and adds to the mystique of his self-analysis. What we cannot see, after all, is much more mysterious than what we can. Were we exposed to all the facts, we might actually feel less persuaded.

A primary function of the myth of his self-analysis now begins to become clear. We have seen that the evidence for the dream as the necessary carrier of the childhood wish in the individual instance is largely allusory and "cannot carry much conviction"; the ubiquity of the wish does not seem to follow inevitably from the data presented. But if another kind of study can be fashioned that is part secret, part legend, and part autobiography, then the dream as the royal road to the past becomes a different and more convincing story. Freud's self-analysis provides us with an experiment in nature, an illustration of his axiom that every dream grows out of a childhood wish. As proof, we have the discoveries about his past that his dreams made possible (and which he partly confirmed by speaking with his mother). If not a demonstration that the axiom is true, his self-analysis at least provides us with suggestive evidence in its support and tends to diminish our initial disbelief. In other words, the myth of his self-analysis takes the issue out of the framework of science and its presumption of hard data and transforms it into the stuff of legend, placing it on a canvas where evidence is no longer at issue.

To fill out this canvas has been the task of Freud's biographers ever since. Each new account has enlarged on and embellished the legend, just as new tellings of the *Odyssey,* in the days before a written version was available, tended to add new adventures to each recital. As pieces of history, the efforts of Freud's biographers are open to question, but as rhetorical achievements that add to the legend of his self-analysis, they are impressive accomplishments, because they come close to convincing us that Freud was able to travel back in time to uncover pieces of his past and to do it almost at will.

If the land of dreams was an unknown continent open to any enterprising explorer, the past was not only a different country but thought to be largely out of reach. What kind of country? From Freud's scattered and largely allusive reports, mainly contained in the letters to Fleiss and thus not intended for publication, we have shadowy glimpses of one or two key figures who never come into clear focus. But this misty island of memories has since been colonized by a new series of explorers—Freud's biographers—who have also, in some remarkable way, been able to travel back in time, land on the same shores, and see farther and more clearly than the original explorer. Each new biographer brings back a new set of discoveries about the mythical self-analysis.

An appropriately respectful tone was first set by Ernest Jones: "In the summer of 1897, the spell began to break and Freud undertook his most heroic feat—a psychoanalysis of his own unconscious. It is hard for us nowadays to imagine how momentous this achievement was, that difficulty being the feat of most pioneering exploits. Yet the uniqueness of the feat remains. Once done it is done forever. For no one again can be the first to explore those depths" (1953, p. 319).

Kurt Eissler is equally eloquent and along similar lines: "The heroism—one is inclined to describe it so—that was necessary to carry out such an undertaking has not yet been sufficiently appreciated. But anyone who has ever undergone a personal analysis will know how strong the impulse is to take flight from insight into the unconscious and the repressed . . . Freud's self-analysis will one day take a place of eminence in the history of ideas, just as the fact that it took place at all will remain, possibly for ever, a problem that is baffling to the psychologist" (1971, pp. 279–280; quoted in Sulloway, 1979, p. 447). The most recent voyager returns in the same spirit. Peter Gay identifies the self-analysis as the "cherished centerpiece of psychoanalytic mythology" and goes on to celebrate "this act of patient heroism, to be admired and palely imitated but never repeated, . . . the founding act of psychoanalysis." And in a later section: "Whatever we call it, Freud in the late 1880s subjected himself to a most thoroughgoing self-scrutiny, *an elaborate, penetrating, and unceasing census* of his fragmentary memories, his concealed wishes and emotions. From tantalizing bits and pieces, he reconstructed fragments of his buried early life, and with the aid of such highly personal reconstructions combined with his clinical experience, sought to sketch the outlines of human nature. He had no precedent for this work, no teachers, but had to invent the rules for it as he went along" (1988, pp. 96–98; italics mine).

The fanciful description of the self-analysis favored by Freud's biographers stands in striking contrast to the scanty evidence available from the Fleiss correspondence and *Die Traumdeutung* and makes us realize all the more that it is his biographers who are mainly responsible for supporting this "centerpiece of psychoanalytic mythology." Each new description adds to its mythical status: Gay's is even more fulsome than Jones's. Each recounting takes pains to point out the "absolute originality" of the feat that is an important aspect of the myth of the hero (see Crews, 1988; Ellenberger, 1970; and Sulloway, 1979). The attempt to carry out the first, last, and only self-analysis (and one might ask, How do we know that it is the only one?) would seem to make its doing more important than its yield. Once again we find that its very vagueness adds to its mystique, allowing it to serve as what Sulloway calls a "heroic vehicle" for Freud's important discoveries. The self-analysis becomes the mandatory "perilous journey" found in all heroic legends. "The story of Freud's heroic self-analysis follows this last archtypical subpattern in many essential respects and may be compared with such equally heroic episodes as Aeneas' descent into the underworld to learn his destiny or Moses' leadership of the Hebrews during the Exodus from Egypt . . . Having undergone his superhuman ordeal, the archtypical hero now emerges as a person transformed, possessing the power to bestow great benefits upon his fellow man" (Sulloway, 1979, p. 447). A parallel description can be found in Crews (1988), who sees psychoanalysis as a story "devised about a mythic Sigismund who had returned from the frightening psychic underworld with precious gifts for humankind" (p. 247).

The beginning of the self-analysis has usually been placed in the summer of 1897 (see Jones, 1953, p. 323; Bonaparte, Freud, and Kris, 1954, p. 211n). In his letter of June 22 of that year, Freud tells Fleiss that he has "been through some kind of a neurotic experience, curious states incomprehensible to [consciousness], twilight thoughts, veiled doubts, with barely a ray of light here or there." In his letter of July 7, he seems to allude to the process and its difficulties: "I know that at the moment I am useless as a correspondent, with no right to any claims, but it was not always so and it will not remain so. *I still do not know what has been happening to me.* Something from the deepest depth of my own neurosis set itself against any advance in the understanding of the neuroses, and you have somehow been involved in it" (Masson, 1985, pp. 254–255; italics mine).

In the ensuing correspondence, there were occasional references to the ongoing analysis and some of its discoveries. In his letter of October 15, Freud promises that "if the [self-] analysis fulfills what I expect of it, I shall work on it systematically and then put it before you." In the same letter, he tells of confirming a reconstruction about his nurse. On October 31 he writes, "My analysis continues and remains my chief interest" (Masson, 1985, p. 272; p. 276).

The promise of October 15 was never fulfilled. The full account of Freud's self-analysis has never been told, and its discoveries are emphasized more by Freud's biographers than by Freud himself. It is more than a little surprising to find no mention of the self-analysis in Freud's autobiography (1925): it is conspicuously missing from both the discussion of infantile sexuality (pp. 33–39) and the summary of *Die Traumdeutung* (pp. 44–46). But the absence of the self-analysis from the official account has not seemed to deter Freud's biographers.

Jones set the heroic tone. Subsequent accounts have elaborated on this model to add other speculations, but the fact remains that the essential details reduce to only a handful of letters (discovered by accident) and some occasional comments in *Die Traumdeutung*. We have no systematic information about the method used, we have only an incomplete account of the important dreams, and we have almost none of the associations, aside from those reported in *Die Traumdeutung*. But the lack of evidence did not stop his biographers from fashioning an extensive myth about its difficulties and its originality, nor from specifying many of its findings (see Sulloway, 1979, Chap. 12, for extended comments on this myth and some of the functions it serves).

With its suggestion of a descent into the underworld, coupled with its associations with a time machine, the legend of Freud's self-analysis cannot help but evoke awe and respect. By surrounding the event with mythic overtones, Freud further increases his authority over the reader. The same could also be said of his biographers. Jones quotes the words of Heraclitus: "The soul of man is a far country, which cannot be approached or explored" (1953, p. 319), only to show that Freud proved him wrong. Not only was Freud an explorer in a distant, untraveled land; he had returned safely from the nether regions. This heroic achievement surrounded even the most passing observation with a kind of final authority. What might be speculation or hypothesis under ordinary circumstances became, against this background of struggle and insight, a conclusion to be carved in stone. We are confronted with a series of authoritative assertions—but assertions tinged with a special mystique that defies counterargument. Specific examples of the rule that infantile wishes are always present in dreams may not be convincing, but these details count for little against the legend of the self-analysis, the insights it yielded and the suffering it entailed.

The suffering is mentioned by each of the biographers and plays a special role in the story by helping to immunize the hero from almost any attack. Faced with this kind of heroic adventure bought at such a price, how can any critic be so unkind as to raise doubts about what it produced? The legend of Freud's self-analysis thus operates as a kind of critical experiment, which silences all criticism and sets a final seal on the achievement. The early discoveries of psychoanalysis become extraordinary achievements bought at great cost and revealed in a mystical and heroic manner that puts them outside the reach of normal science. So runs the rhetorical message.

Against this mythical background, the specific rhetorical figures used by Freud take on additional power. Argument by authority becomes, as we have seen, a voice from on high (or from the depths, if we believe that he carried out some kind of underworld exploration). The fallacy of generalizing from a single case loses much of its force once the single case has acquired heroic stature. Freud is no longer one man among many but a special kind of explorer endowed with mythical powers and possessed of extraordinary insight. His self-analysis, this one-of-a-kind expedition into the unconscious and into the past, would seem to exempt him from the normal constraints of science, freeing him to make extreme statements without fear of challenge, to invoke unspecified observations in support of his conclusions, and to mimimize the need for replication and validation.

Freud himself seemed well aware of the fact that pure ideas speak in low voices and often go unheard. He was constantly adding a rhetorical flourish that would translate the idea into a personal statement and give his theory a more direct appeal. In a letter to Fliess on June 12, 1900, Freud allows himself to fantasize about Bellevue, the summer house where he had analyzed the famous specimen dream some five years before. "Do you suppose," he writes, "that someday one will read a marble tablet on this house: 'Here, on July 24, 1895, the secret of the dream revealed itself to Dr. Sigm. Freud.' So far there is little prospect of it" (Masson, 1985, p. 417). And in an earlier letter, Freud ironically describes himself as "the author of the 'extremely important book on dreams, which unfortunately is not yet sufficiently appreciated by scientists' " (Masson, 1985, p. 358).

In a related attempt to generalize from the theory of dreams to a somewhat broader domain of discourse, Freud used as his epigraph for *Die Traumdeutung* a line from the *Aeneid:* "Flectere si nequeo superos, Acheronta movebo" (If I cannot bend the Higher Powers, I will move the Infernal Regions). Conquest of the unconscious becomes linked to doing battle with the devil, and in the process, the emerging theory acquires religious and supernatural overtones. Critics of the theory now become associated with its enemies—the underworld and the devil. As a result, any rival author is automatically viewed with suspicion, and believed to be in league with the dark powers and resistant to the Truth.

Freud's mythic standing tempts biographers to endow him with even greater glory and to assign him attributes he may not have possessed. Thus, Gay tells us that "Freud did not regard his own experiences as automatically valid for all humanity. He tested his notions against the experiences of his patients and, later, against the psychoanalytic literature; he spent years working over, refining, revising, his generalizations" (1988, p. 90). But because Gay cites no source for this laudatory conclusion, we begin to suspect that it is yet another piece of the myth of the hero. Indeed, the facts of the matter suggest quite the opposite. Once Freud had made up his mind, he was unusually resistant to changing it. Far from being concerned with replication, Freud was less than gracious to his critics and tended to look on counterarguments as a challenge to his authority and a suspicious sign of loss of trust.

Further additions to the hero myth can be found in Gay's account of Freud's self-revelations: "Though intent on maintaining his privacy and averse to disclosing his inner life to strangers, he yielded [sic] to the pressure, for the sake of science, to be indiscreet about himself" (1988, p. 90). But the pressure did not come from science; it came from the need to persuade others of the rightness of his views. He could not use clinical material from his patients because he needed to protect their privacy and because they were mentally ill; their pathology, it could be argued, must necessarily affect their thought processes. To build the foundation of a general psychology, Freud had to show the workings of a normal dreamer, and for that purpose, he needed to present his own dreams.

Secrecy as a Rhetorical Device

It is worth commenting on the secrecy surrounding Freud's self-analysis and how that feature has worked in Freud's favor. The use of secrecy as what might be called a rhetorical device has a long history in early science, and it led in part to the revolutionary efforts of Bacon and his colleagues to put science once and for all in the public domain. The influence of the occult sciences during the Middle Ages was heightened by their secrecy and by the fact that they were not public knowledge but confined to a small circle of insiders. As a result, it was not always apparent whether an authority was telling the truth. Two kinds of alchemists were identified:

> An alchemist is said to be *grudging* if he knowingly gives wrong information about his Art, and *generous* if he reveals a truth. So one of the first things a student has to learn is to recognize whether an alchemical work comes from the pen of a *grudging* author or from one who is *generous,* and it is no use hoping that he will ever be able to distinguish them by rule of thumb. In the main, there are two kinds of books on alchemy—those in which the writer says that he is convinced of the futility of alchemical speculations and therefore that the creation of the Philosopher's Stone is an impossibility; and those in which the author, introducing himself as an "amateur" . . .

says that he is bound by the traditional vow of secrecy, and therefore that any revelations about substances or processes used in the Work are not only worthless but actually dangerous. (Sadoul, 1972, p. 213)

Whereas the "new science" of the seventeenth century was pledged to a tradition of open investigation and public findings, a different set of rules seems to apply to Freud's self-analysis. Rather than question its yield and conclude from its very vagueness that it was not a significant factor, Freud's biographers (including even the generally critical Sulloway) are all impressed by the mystery of the undertaking and even find the secrecy to be one of its virtues. We can see its appeal for the biographer. When next to nothing is known about a topic, the biographer's hand is freed and he writes with no fear of contradiction. Future voyages to this mysterious island will undoubtedly bring back even more fantastic and detailed reports; even as it sinks further into the past, its specifics somehow become clearer and clearer. In valorizing the mystery of the undertaking and showing themselves to be more pleased than sorry by the absence of hard fact, the consumers of the self-analysis legend would seem to belong more to the pre-Renaissance tradition of conceptualist science than to the modern Baconian tradition.

Secrecy was also useful for another reason. The self-analysis is regularly invoked as the source of many of Freud's most innovative ideas, and its very vagueness makes it all the easier to assert this claim. Commentators have discovered in his self-analysis the reasons for the "abandonment of the seduction theory and . . . his discoveries of infantile sexuality, the Oedipus complex, the theory of dreams, the free association technique, the concepts of transference and resistance, and even the unconscious" (Sulloway, 1979, p. 207). Ernst Kris is among the most explicit of this group: "The first and perhaps most significant result of Freud's self-analysis was the step from the seduction theory to full insight into the significance of infantile sexuality" (Bonaparte, Freud, and Kris, 1954, p. 33). Although Sulloway is skeptical—"the decision to abandon the seduction theory was the culmination of a long conceptual transformation, influenced much more by Fliess and by the inherent flaws of the seduction theory itself than by self-analysis" (1979, p. 208)—he is one of the very few critics. For most readers, the self-analysis remains the fountainhead of psychoanalysis.

Given the meager documentation that supports it, Freud's self-analysis lends itself to any number of explanations with no fear of contradiction. It not only serves as a possible source for many of Freud's ideas, it also provides an excellent means of bridging the gap between Freud's Zeitgeist—particularly his conventional scientific training—and his innovative theory. And it shelters his more unusual ideas from the demand for evidence. While we may never know the precise relationship between the self-analysis and the development of psychoanalytic theory, it becomes more convincing to invoke the self-analysis as a source of a particular concept (such as the Oedipus complex) than to concede that this complex was only one of Freud's more idiosyncratic ideas. We begin to see why the self-analysis is so frequently invoked as an explanation, despite its rather shadowy standing.

But while Freud's theory, according to this line of reasoning, was based on evidence (the revelations of the self-analysis), its contents (aside from the scattered references in his letters and occasional allusions in his writings) are not open to public inspection. This is evidence of a rather peculiar kind. It is therefore significant that so much importance has been attributed to this one source, an illustration once again of the influence of the Aristotelian tradition. What is more, the frequent dependence on secrecy is not an isolated instance in the history of psychoanalysis. Heavy reliance on secret sources has continued to characterize (and plague) psychoanalysis up to the present time. Consider the role of early experience on later development, the impact of early memories on later behavior, and the role of the clinical happening on the published report. As Jacobsen and Steele (1979) have pointed out, Freud "begins with observations of adult pathology and moves from the adult present via psychoanalytic interpretations to the infantile past. This past is then considered to be real and contain within it causes for the present" (p. 353). But because it is set in some earlier time period, the triggering event can never be inspected directly; thus the hypothesis can never be tested directly.

Not only is this pattern of looking for distant causes in present events a common occurrence in psychoanalytic reasoning, it is also recognized as one of its standard rhetorical figures, formally known as *metalepsis*. Defined as attributing a present effect to a remote cause, this figure has been described as "a kinde of Metonymie, signifying by the effect a Cause far off by an effect nigh at hand. [It] teaches the understanding to dive down to the bottom of the sense, and instructs the eye of the wit to discern a meaning afar off" (Smith, 1657; cited in Vickers, 1988, p. 331). This figure has become an established part of psychoanalytic explanations, and we will meet it again in Chapter 6. One of the first times it was used came about when Freud decided to *allude* to the insights of his self-analysis but never bring the details into the public domain. (We must bear in mind that if the Fliess letters had not been discovered, the self-analysis would never have come up for discussion).

By keeping the self-analysis screened from public view, Freud managed to increase its mythic status and make it possible for others in the psychoanalytic community to endow it with whatever content they wish. We have already seen some evidence of this projection in the quotations from Jones and Gay, and we can assume that the unpublished fantasies of other commentators and analysts are equally mythic in their connotations. Once concealed from view, this feat quickly began to acquire mythical overtones, and it can be argued that once the legend began to build, it became impossible to publish the real thing—the actual findings would be too disappointing. This may have been one reason why Freud never published his notebooks.

When Freud wrote about his self-analysis, was he being *grudging* or *generous* (the distinction made in the occult tradition quoted above)? His biographers fail to appreciate the difference and apparently believe that his comments to Fleiss and his allusions in *Die Traumdeutung* can be given as much credence as the texts of his dreams. Jones was more than ready to believe the full account: "Freud told me [that] he never ceased to analyze himself, devoting the last half hour of his day to that purpose. One more example of his flawless integrity" (1953, p. 327). In recognition of this undocumented claim, Jones titles the chapter "Self-Analysis (1897–)," the missing date telling us that it continued throughout his life. Gay repeats the same claim: Even though "there are vital details of Freud's self-analysis that are likely to remain obscure . . . he doubtless conducted it every day [how do we know?] . . ." Gay is uncertain only as to the details: "Did he take what free time he had in the evening, or did he analyze himself at slack times during consulting hours? Did he pursue his intense, often dismaying ruminations when he took his early afternoon walk to rest from his posture as the professional listener and to buy his cigars? This much we know" (1988, p. 98). Gay is taking a leaf from Freud's own rhetorical manual; he not only uses the voice of authority ("this much we know") to convince the reader, he also relies on the trope of enargia, adding details (afternoon walk, buying cigars) in order to lend verisimilitude to the incident and take attention away from the possibility that it is essentially only speculation and may never have happened in this way at all. The fact of the matter is that we have no documentation of the regularity, the method used, or the specific accumulation of insights, and we may easily wonder whether the overall account should not be seen as one of Freud's more *grudging* admissions.

A similar conclusion can be drawn from the Preface to the second edition of *Traumdeutung* (written in 1908 and reprinted in the *Standard Edition*). It is more than a little disturbing to find Freud remarking, "I am glad to say that I have found little to change . . . Here and there I have inserted some new material, added some fresh points of detail derived from my increased experience, and at some few points recast my statements. But the *essence of what I have written about dreams and their interpretation . . . remains unaltered: subjectively at all events, it has stood the test of time*" (1900, p. xxv; italics mine).

This statement can hardly be true. At the least, it puts the lie to Gay's optimistic belief that Freud "spent years working over, refining, revising his generalizations" (1988, p. 90), or Jones's claim that Freud was possessed by an "overpowering need to come at the truth at all costs, [a need that] was probably the deepest and strongest motive force in Freud's personality, one to which everything else—ease, success, happiness—must be sacrificed" (1953, p. 320). We may choose to discount his biographers' more rhapsodic statements, but we cannot overlook the fact that the early findings of any new domain of investigation are almost invariably revised as more evidence comes to light. While writing the first edition of *Die Traumdeutung*, Freud was bringing a new theory into view for the first time, and although many of its hypotheses may have been overstated, as we have seen, they could still be taken as sincere. But after almost ten years of clinical experience (and, according to Jones and Gay, a day-by-day continuation of his self-analysis), it seems highly unlikely that essentially all of the formulations could survive unchanged.

Rather than accept the second edition Preface as evidence for the basic soundness of his theory, it seems more reasonable to read it as a sign that Freud had moved closer to the traditions of conceptualist science and was taking a stand against the principles of the new empiricists. Contrary to the new science of Bacon and his followers, findings are not to be replicated until they meet some public standard; the law of large numbers can be set aside in favor of unparalleled insight. It is his self-analysis that allows Freud to set himself outside the post-Renaissance scientific tradition and claim special privileges in gaining access to, and making interpretations of, the evidence. And it is his self-analysis that gives his biographers permission to exempt him from the expectations of normal science. There is another reason why it looms so large in the standard biography of Freud: it gives his biographers the license to accentuate the more unusual discoveries without having to account for their sources and to describe his development as a theorist without having to explain many of the contradictions implicit in his history.

Its Place in the Conceptualist Tradition

Additional functions served by Freud's self-analysis come to light when we consider it from the perspective of Aristotelian science. We have seen that penetrating knowledge of the specimen is available only to the qualified observer. As a result, his insights are privileged and those who lack similar qualifications must give way before his authority. His self-analysis stamps Freud as the *only* expert qualified to understand the link between adult dreams and infantile wishes. It is entirely in keeping with the tradition of medieval science to accept his testimony as final. Freud's biographers (and, to a large extent, his followers) are influenced, wittingly or unwittingly, by the same tradition. One would expect Gay's experience as a historian to make him look suspiciously at the documentation for both the doing and the outcome of the self-analysis, yet he unhesitatingly accepts the fact that it took place just as Jones and Freud say it did. Freud's authority goes unquestioned.

Not only did the skilled follower of Aristotelian science find the specimen "essentially transparent and therefore completely intelligible," but he was able, on account of his special talents, to find universal principles in the singular object (McMullin, 1967, p. 333). It becomes consistent with conceptualist science to conclude that penetrating knowledge of the specimen in question—Freud's unconscious—could allow him to uncover the essential principles of the new science. Gay's summary of the self-analysis legend parallels almost exactly the defining language of conceptualist science. Where Gay tells us that Freud "sought to sketch the outline of human nature" from "an elaborate, penetrating and unceasing census of his fragmentary memories, his concealed wishes and emotions" (1988, p. 97), McMullin grounds conceptualist science on the "insight on the part of a skilled investigator into the singular object of sense . . . sufficiently penetrating to allow the universal to be immediately grasped" (1967, p. 333). Once the self-analysis has been accepted as the "founding act of psychoanalysis" (Gay, 1988, p. 96), the medieval scientist (and contemporary psychoanalyst) would find it logical to assume that any number of sound principles could be derived from it.

From the standpoint of conceptualist science, the self-analysis becomes the keystone of the whole structure. It warrants Freud's status as the supremely qualified investigator whose judgment must be accepted without question, it suggests a natural origin for many of the theory's more challenging and nonintuitive assumptions, and it shows clearly the importance of the Aristotelian tradition. Given the grounding assumptions of this tradition, it seems only natural to privilege one man's opinions over those of his peers, to remain unconcerned by the absence of evidence (for either the self-analysis or the central propositions of the theory), and to remain untroubled by the problem of individual differences and the possibility that Freud's observations might not apply to everyone. These questions simply do not present themselves to the Aristotelian scientist, and so long as he can return to the self-analysis as the primary specimen, he has no difficulty accepting the rest of the theory. Freud's biographers may have sensed what a crucial role it plays in grounding the theory in an established tradition and perhaps for this reason have successively embellished and romanticized the legend.

If psychoanalysis could claim membership in the conceptualist tradition, then it was further protected from standard empiricist challenges. Failure to observe the law of large numbers, absence of systematic replication, problems of generalizability, and all the other standard criticisms of new discoveries would seem not to apply because Freud's findings were uncovered by another route. Thus the self-analysis provides all-around protection despite its many flaws. These flaws, as I noted earlier, stem from the disproportion of rhetoric to evidence and the suspicion that Freud's biographers have been more enthusiastic than systematic. But even this form of criticism belongs more to our present tradition than to the arguments of conceptualist science. Because the principal complaints come from a different universe of discourse, their impact is significantly muted—which may explain why psychoanalysis has survived for so long without any significant changes.

Its inexplicable survival has long perplexed critics of psychoanalysis, who often find themselves wondering, in varied degrees of exasperation, how this longevity can be explained. Here is a typical complaint:

> As someone who spent a decade inching his way from a pro-psychoanalytic stance to an opposite one, I am more than usually aware that Freudianism is internally resilient against exposure of its implausibility. The resilience lies not in intellectual virtues possessed by the theory but in the nature of its appeal to its adherents . . . Indeed, as many observers have noted, psychoanalysis shows every sign of being not just a method and a psychology but also a faith, with all that this implies about psychic immunity from rationally based criticism. Like other faiths, Freudianism readily rebounds when confronted with seemingly fatal objections, for its believers have rendered it inseparable from their private sense of spiritual vitality and worth. (Crews, 1988, p. 236)

One reason for this resilience may lie in the Aristotelian tradition. Just as it protects Freud from his enemies and safeguards him from the checks and balances of normal science, so it also protects the early findings against the charge that they have not been sufficiently replicated, that they are based on too small a number of cases, that much of the argument has not been supported by evidence, and that much of the little evidence we have is secret and therefore not open to public inspection. Even well-founded critiques tend to disappear from view soon after publication. Grünbaum's *The Foundations of Psychoanalysis,* first published in 1984 to largely welcoming reviews, was cited only three times in the 1992 volume of the *Journal of the American Psychoanalytic Association.* It was cited in Gay's recent biography (1988) but not directly confronted or extensively discussed. Hobson's rival theory of dreams (1988) has had a similar fate; it was cited only twice in the same volume of the same journal. At least two explanations for this absence of influence suggest themselves. First, neither of these critiques was preceded by a one-of-a-kind self-analysis, subsequently buttressed by historians and biographers. Second, the books come from a different tradition of scholarship than *Die Traumdeutung* and as a result fall largely on deaf ears. (Hanly's review of Grünbaum points out that "Grünbaum is an inductivist in the tradition of Bacon and Mill . . . Grünbaum would have no criticism of psychoanalysis if he thought that psychoanalytic clinical observations had the probative value of Galileo's telescopic observations of the moon's surface . . . or of Harvey's experiment that established the circulation of the blood . . . The Achilles' heel of Grünbaum's argument is his failure to understand the nature of the analytic process" [1988, pp. 524–526]).

A closer look at *Foundations of Psychoanalysis* will show in more detail where some of the differences lie. A large section of Grünbaum's book is given over to a critique of free association as an investigatory procedure. These comments have received almost no attention from the profession, and the explanation may be the fact that the *method* of free association is of little interest apart from its findings. It is common knowledge that in the proper hands (Freud's in particular), the method is useful; thus there is little reason to discuss it further. As we saw in Chapter 3, method in the Aristotelian tradition is clearly secondary to the specimen—exactly the opposite of the assumptions of Galilean science. Bacon and his colleagues at the Royal Society were dedicated to the belief that science was an essentially democratic enterprise. They assumed that once the method was clearly described, the particular example was not important. Psychoanalysis falls back on an earlier tradition, which highlights the specimen by putting it first, the investigator (his standing determined by his talents and qualifications) next, and method last. Because method is a distant third, it is never discussed in isolation from its application (we might recall the secrecy surrounding the procedures used by the alchemists to extract gold from lead).

After pointing to the difficulties adhering to free association as a general method for gathering clinical data and referring in particular to the extent to which the data are corrupted by the patient's wish to please the analyst, Grünbaum goes on to suggest that the basic principles of psychoanalysis may perhaps be true but require extra-clinical validation before they can be generally accepted as part of normal science. But extra-clinical validation using the methods of empiricist science not only presupposes an entirely new and different set of validating principles; in proposing such a procedure, Grünbaum is implicitly challenging the assumptions of Aristotelian science. If the old ways must be given up, then the full range of privileged specimens—the Dora case, the Irma dream, Freud's self-analysis, and similar clinical happenings—must be exchanged for a new set of investigations using different rules, and the outcome of these studies is still very much in doubt. To give up these specimens is, furthermore, to put an end to the possibility of cumulative discovery, building on what has already been found. Who is to say what further insights may come to light? Who would exchange the Dora case for an unexamined clinical happening?

By proposing extra-clinical validation of the fundamental concepts of psychoanalysis, Grünbaum is, in effect, dismissing the Aristotelian tradition that has been fundamental to both the theory and practice of psychoanalysis. He may feel that this tradition has been bankrupt ever since the Renaissance and was superseded by something finer, but this opinion is less than persuasive to the average analyst, who tends to see the world as made up of a series of wondrous specimens, each waiting to be interpreted, and who is concerned more with specific examples than with general laws. Trained to believe that some investigators (practitioners or supervisors) are more skilled than others and to respect secrecy as a necessary part of their profession, he sees no reason to challenge Freud's superiority as the first analyst and father of psychoanalytic theory. Believers in Freud's self-analysis as the fountainhead of the basic discoveries, these practitioners cannot help but be heartened by the sympathetic embellishments of Jones, Eissler, and Gay. They have no reason to be skeptical because their sense of what happened during the self-analysis coincides more or less exactly with the biographers' most romantic version. Because the concept of privileged observer possessed with penetrating wisdom not available to the average investigator forms so important a part of the conceptualist tradition, questions of subjective bias or observer error never emerge. All versions of the self-analysis highlight Freud's role as the innovative explorer of unknown regions, and because this image meshes so well with the traditional conceptualist view of science, the biographers' version is immediately accepted as fact.

We now begin to understand another side of the Aristotelian tradition. Grounded in the detailed description of privileged specimens, it is more responsive to rhetoric than to logic, to words than to numbers. New accounts of Freud's self-analysis cannot fail to hold everyone's attention because they deepen the romance that already surrounds this adventure and promise new insights into Freud's descent into (and return from) the dark regions of the mind. But methodological criticisms such as those mounted by Grünbaum and, before him, by Nagel (1959) and Hook (1959), are speaking from another tradition, which honors method over investigator and abstract principles over concrete examples. Grünbaum, Nagel, and Hook are not necessarily in error; they have simply made the mistake of adopting the wrong paradigm and for that reason remain largely unheard.

We can now extend the answer to the question that puzzled Crews and has perplexed even more sympathetic critics. Psychoanalysis survives in significant measure because its practitioners can identify with the Aristotelian tradition, which gives selected authorities permission to choose specimen objects for study, draw conclusions from these specimens, and expand these conclusions into theory. The tradition honors the study of single examples—symptoms, cases, or therapeutic hours—and penetrating knowledge of these examples can be used to generate universal principles. This tradition allows fact-finding to be delegated to a select few, ultimately chosen on the basis of either their clinical expertise or their association with acknowledged experts in the course of training, supervision, or control analyses. (It is one of the special features of psychoanalysis that clinical acumen becomes the accepted basis for scientific competence).

To the extent that this tradition celebrates the good example as the ultimate source of knowledge, it tends to focus attention on landmark cases, specimen dreams, and one-of-a-kind clinical examples. It therefore should come as no surprise to find that Freud's self-analysis has been so enthusiastically celebrated and that subsequent accounts of it are treated almost as replications. What is being replicated, of course, is not a set of data but the sense, common to any great myth, that *this* is the way things happened and that, once again, agony, pain, and suffering are small prices to pay when the reward is so great. Given this kind of reading, it is no wonder that rhetorical embellishments are largely overlooked and that even an experienced historian like Gay is only too willing to silence his skepticism and add his account to the rest. The race is on to see who can craft the most compelling adventure.

If Freud's self-analysis is seen as the centerpiece, capstone, and fountainhead of standard theory, then it automatically becomes the primary specimen. In keeping with conceptualist beliefs, we stand to learn more from repeated study of this legend—the Rosetta Stone of psychoanalysis—than from gathering new data. This particular specimen is privileged because we know its credentials, we acknowledge that both analyst (Freud) and patient (Freud) are above reproach, and we already have proof that some of its insights have yielded universal laws. Nothing is to be lost by repeated investigation of the specimen and much may be gained. But an investigation of more recent clinical happenings—that strikes the traditional conceptualist as a much more doubtful undertaking. How do we know, first of all, that the new specimen will reveal its secrets? For that to happen, the investigator must be clearly qualified as a supreme clinician, a product of only the finest institutes, and have a long string of clinical successes to his credit. If he is not a clearly privileged investigator, then the specimen will never become transparent and nothing of interest will be discovered.

Some Implications

Up to this point, I have been attempting to show the relevance of Freud's self-analysis for the Aristotelian scientist and how, from that point of view, its emphasis on rhetoric over evidence seems quite natural and unexceptional. But from the standpoint of twentieth-century science, we must take a rather different position. If the self-analysis is more rhetoric than history, then it can no longer be used as the centerpiece of psychoanalysis and an example of the penetrating analysis of the specimen so necessary for conceptualist science. And if such an analysis never took place in the manner described (in a fashion dictated by the conceptualist tradition), then we are less certain about whether Freud can claim to be the *only* authority, whether his view is any more penetrating than that of his critics, or whether the universals discovered in this particular specimen have any particular validity.

If the self-analysis is more rhetoric than history, then we are still waiting for the skeptical biographer who finds himself able to stand outside the Jones-Eissler-Gay tradition and tell a less romantic story. Such a biographer must be able to resist adding his own embellishments to the myth of the hero. If he were able to demonstrate this kind of fortitude, he would probably be in a position to write a more faithful account, because once the biographer falls under the spell of the self-analysis legend, he becomes captive to all the other aspects of the psychoanalytic tradition. Once he agrees with Jones that this momentous achievement was Freud's "most heroic feat" and with Gay that "this act of patient heroism has never been repeated," he is hostage to the movement. Once he concedes the sacrifice and suffering necessary to carry out this task, he is in no position to criticize the quality of the evidence or the nature of the conclusions.

The same rule also applies to the reader. If he can read the self-analysis as a mixture of history and rhetoric and be properly skeptical at the places where the evidence grows faint, then he shows an awareness of the power of the rhetorical voice and defines himself as a reliable consumer of Freud's style. But if he finds each new telling of the legend to be an improvement over the last, then he makes it clear that he has placed himself in the hands of a master story-teller and that from that point on, he will probably be unable to read Freud in a properly critical fashion. The *Standard Edition* then becomes a sacred text. Such is the power of rhetoric, which can, as Nehamas says, "subordinate knowledge to action and reason to will" (1988, p. 771).

The self-analysis legend also interferes with a careful and systematic reassessment of the theory, and here is where its largely rhetorical message creates the most mischief. So long as the origin of Freud's theory is hidden inside a secret and mysterious set of events that will never be fully reconstructed, the conclusions springing from these events are above reproach and beyond criticism. The myth of Freud's self-analysis provides psychoanalysis with an unassailable birthright, and it is the staying power of this myth that makes the theory so hard to criticize, enabling it to persevere in the face of doubtful evidence. Because all the important features of the theory can be found in the discoveries of Freud's self-analysis, criticism of almost any kind is quickly seen as ungrateful and ill-mannered, the behavior of someone who, incredibly enough, does not know what the self-analysis cost in pain and suffering. If Freud analyzed himself during a part of every day for almost forty years, goes the argument, how can someone who knows nothing of this experience find the nerve to find fault? We are back to a conceptualist position once again: the untrained observer must defer to the recognized authority, for it is only through his wisdom that we can learn to read the world.

6 The Misleading Case Study

When Freud ended his work with Dora, he told a friend that he had just finished writing an account so exciting that coming out from under its spell, he felt "short of a drug" (that is, as if he were suffering from withdrawal symptoms; see Klein and Tribich, 1982, p. 14). To this day, the case report remains our most compelling means of communicating clinical findings, and the excitement attached to both reading and writing case histories has lost none of its appeal. Freud's early clinical discussions continue to be studied and restudied, and the form of presentation he developed so well—the classical narrative presentation—still influences the way we present our clinical discoveries. But as we look at this tradition from a more detached perspective, we begin to find flaws in the method and can identify significant changes in the way it is practiced.

Over the past one hundred years, the ratio of detail to narrative has tended to decline. Where specific clinical vignettes and near-verbatim dreams can be found in both Freud's Dora and Wolf Man cases, to name only two examples, today's reader would be hard pressed to find a current case that contains a comparable amount of specific information. Verbatim dreams tend to be the exception rather than the rule, and verbatim dialogue is almost never presented. Even when verbatim material is offered, it is not always clear how much selection and/or revision has taken place. As a result, the reader has little chance to make direct contact with the clinical data and arrive at his own conclusions independent of the opinion of the treating analyst. Moreover, because the description of the clinical happening is almost never presented in its original form, it becomes all the more difficult to separate observation from inference or data from theory.

118

Without direct access to the clinical data, the reader is deprived of the chance to use what Isakower has called the "analyzing instrument" (Balter, Lothane, and Spencer, 1980). This instrument has been developed through years of clinical training and experience to read between the lines, to generate multiple accounts of specific clinical happenings, and to be exquisitely tolerant of ambiguity. To apply such an instrument to a finished narrative that is largely devoid of the kind of detail analysts use in making clinical inferences becomes a frustrating and unsatisfying exercise that tends to deprive the reader of the opportunity to compare his own thinking with that of the author's. He is thus excluded from joining a dialogue in which the intricacies of clinical process and findings can be more fully and definitively explored.

Problems arise in psychoanalytic discourse as a result of its undue reliance on anecdote, aggravated by the understandable tendency of the writer to select material that supports his position. Anecdotal case reports tend to highlight clinical observations that conform to expectations, and thus to confirm accepted theory. Such reports reduce the opportunity for surprise by omitting the unique or unexpected event, yet it is precisely these surprises that may generate a good part of our clinical wisdom. When detail is omitted, the interpretations of the treating analyst are prone to be accepted as the final decision: the "privileged competence" of the treating analyst (Spence, 1982) is often judged to be sufficient for understanding the clinical happening fully. Writing within this case tradition, the author/analyst may feel no need to reveal all the details of a particular event, assuming that an anecdotal report is sufficient to indicate the general point. But we all know that different analysts listen in different ways and, starting with the same clinical material, often arrive at different conclusions. Because there are many ways of viewing a particular clinical happening, we often need more extensive data to form our judgments. Hence we should ask for supporting evidence whenever possible.

What are the risks of assuming that the author is in the best position to decide what to include or delete in the way of supporting clinical material? A narrative report is necessarily selective, but these selections may be arbitrary or conform to a set of established principles. Even if we agree with the general belief that selective reporting is unavoidable, we begin to realize that not all omissions are equal. Interesting and significant details (including even the patient's initial diagnosis) that might change the thinking of some readers and influence their conclusions are often omitted. So long as there is no indication of what has been left out or changed, the reader must necessarily rely on the authority of the presenter and remain unsure about the accuracy of the information.

We can summarize the changes in case reporting by saying that the current literature tends to emphasize the *necessary* truths found in the clinical happening, whereas earlier case studies tended to emphasize *contingent* truths. In the formative years of psychoanalysis, the investigator could not fall back on general laws and relied on an accumulation of details to persuade the reader of the truthfulness of his account. This reliance on Geertz's "thick description" is very much dependent, as we have seen, on the rhetorical figure of enargia; it uses the concrete immediacy of the here-and-now to convey the sense of hard reality. As psychoanalysis aspired to becoming more of a Galilean science, the clinical particularity was exchanged for this or that "covering law." But because the instantiation of the law was usually less than satisfactory, received theory was given more reinforcement than it deserved, and an interesting exception to the law was never reported in full.

Another way of describing the change in reporting style is to say that reliance on the correspondence theory of truth took precedence over the coherence theory. When explanation is grounded in the coherence theory, an accumulation of detail is required to bring about persuasion because it is only by an account of the relationship among the particular parts of a happening that an explanation can be critically evaluated. But when we turn to correspondence theory, the need for detailed reporting is significantly reduced.

When detail is exchanged for covering law, the language changes as well. If reliance on the best example was the only way to carry the argument and persuade the reader, the intricacies of the clinical happening—the target specimen—were necessarily described in painstaking detail. Deprived of mathematics (or other general, abstract systems) as a form of discourse, Freud concentrated on careful accounts of specimen cases. These accounts were laced with rhetorical figures because of his wish to convey, as clearly as possible, the particularity of the clinical happening in a way that would make it come alive for the reader. If the argument is best framed in terms of contingent truths, then the account *must* be open to the full range of details that constitute the specimen under study. To capture this interweaving of meanings is a classical rhetorical task.

As Freud became more comfortable with the rhetorical power of the case study genre, he began to create increasingly persuasive clinical vignettes. His five classic cases have been praised as "rare works of art and a record of the human mind in one of its most unparalleled works of scientific discovery" (Kanzer and Glenn, 1980). The case method has been described as the "only possible way of obtaining the granite blocks of data on which to build a science of human nature" (Murray, 1955; both sources cited in Runyan, 1982). But as his approach became more widely practiced, a troubling change in both form and content began to take shape. Where Freud might report the verbatim text of one or more of his patient's dreams, subsequent analysts began to rely more and more on paraphrase and summary to convey important clinical material. Where Freud might attempt a near-verbatim reproduction of a significant interchange with a patient, subsequent analysts would report only the themes discussed and withhold the clinical particulars. As a result of the increasing reliance on anecdote and paraphrase to tell the clinical story, the curious reader was often unable to find the specific detail he needed to feel persuaded. When clinical particulars were not presented, the skeptical reader found himself unable to learn exactly how a specific interpretation came about or whether a specific clinical opening might have been followed by an alternative interpretation.

These changes in reporting style have led to the modern case report and to what might be called its "closed" texture. Barring a handful of well-publicized exceptions, the typical case report has only a single story to tell, and it tends to tell it with heavy reliance on anecdote and narrative persuasion and with a preference for what might be called singular explanation. (Freud also shared some of these faults, but they were mitigated by his fondness for archival detail. Today's authors amplify the problem by continuing the singular explanation and omitting most of the significant particulars.)

The singular solution has become an expected part of our clinical tradition. Clinical interchanges are almost always presented as if the interpretation proposed were the only interpretation possible, as if the formulation of the case were the only conceivable formulation, dictated inexorably by the clinical material (which is often conspicuous by its absence). This tradition makes for enjoyable, even fascinating reading but seriously interferes with anyone, either in our time or in future generations, who would like to use the data in ways other than those chosen by the author. The open texture of the clinical happenings is simply not represented by the closed nature of the argument.

Also worth noting is the fact that the facts within the typical case report are almost always seen within a positivistic frame. The observer/therapist is almost always separated from the object/patient being studied. The facts are as concrete and unambiguous as the patient's height and weight and a good deal less ambiguous than his heart sounds or the quality of his resting pulse. Facts in the case study are knowable pieces of reality "out there," distinct as to size and shape, guiding us inevitably in one direction or the other. While the effect of countertransference on our judgments of the clinical situation is more and more being called into question, these considerations have not, to date, materially affected the nature of the case report. Where the clinical reality, as we are coming to realize, is in actuality quite ambiguous and multiply-determined, the facts in the usual clinical account are signposts or barometer readings that lead us unerringly to the solution. We are gradually coming to learn that many of these so-called "facts" are created by us, that they never exist until we choose to see or hear the clinical encounter in a particular way, and that without the perspective of the treating therapist, they can easily be misinterpreted and might even disappear.

A third feature of the case study genre that deserves critical attention is the tradition of argument by authority. The evidence is never so complete that we, as readers, can draw our own conclusions about the clinical happenings; we must therefore give way to the views of the author/analyst. But this tradition seriously interferes with the possibility of friendly disagreement; it tends to support the tradition of privileged withholding (about which I will have more to say in a moment) and takes a position that differs in significant ways from the prevailing scientific Zeitgeist. Argument by authority stands in the way of open disagreement and of the benefits, zealously guarded since the Renaissance, of an adversarial, critical, and dialectical tradition of investigation. We now see that the closed texture of the case report effectively cuts off disagreement because only the author has access to all the facts; thus the author's report is always privileged. But we also know that the first reading of a clinical happening is rarely the last and that certain kinds of understanding only emerge from extended discussion, open disagreement, and spirited challenges to this or that assumption. Thus the nature of the case study, as it is usually practiced, tends to stand in the way of understanding through dialogue and to violate our clinical experience, which has sensitized us to ways in which understanding changes over time.

The problem of privileged withholding has two aspects. On the one hand, we are sensitive to the need to protect the private life of the patient and we disguise pertinent details in an effort to carry out this aim. On the other, if somewhat less in our awareness as authors, is the need to protect ourselves. As a result of either or both of these influences, case reports tend to exclude the very details of the treatment from which we have the most to learn. In carrying out both kinds of disguise, we would seem to be breaking a central clinical rule and going against years of acquired clinical experience. Freud taught us the lesson early in his practice: "I once treated a high official who was bound by his oath of office not to communicate certain things because they were state secrets, and the analysis came to grief as a consequence of this restriction." The reason is clear: "It is very remarkable how the whole task becomes impossible if a reservation is allowed at any single place. But we have only to reflect what would happen if the right of asylum existed at any one point in a town; how long would it be before all the riffraff of the town had collected there" (1913, p. 136).

The permission to tell less than the full story (which Freud granted once and, we assume, never again) is extended all the time to authors of clinical cases—that is, to all publishing analysts. By giving the author of a case report the right to tell less than the complete story, we break rules for ourselves that we would never break for our patients.

Because the case study is our primary means of reporting clinical happenings, the defects of the case study genre have important implications for the progress of psychoanalysis as a science. If the case study tends to be anecdotal and selective, consciously and unconsciously self-serving, and biased toward a singular solution, it can be seen that our literature is seriously incomplete. Not only are we being continuously deprived of salient facts, but the facts reported and the interpretations placed on them tend to conform to the prevailing Zeitgeist, since the case study genre tends to inflate the status of prevailing theory. This state of affairs comes about because of the tendency of the case report to make highly visible the clinical happenings that seem to mesh with received theory and to underplay, or exclude entirely, those happenings that cannot be explained, that go against theoretical understanding, or that result in bad therapeutic outcomes. It is well known that reports of terminated but unsuccessful analyses are significantly hard to find.

We now begin to realize why psychoanalytic theory as we know it today is relatively undifferentiated from Freud's original conception. Studies supporting the received theory are more readily understood and, for that reason, more readily turned into narrative reports. These reports, because they mesh with the prevailing Zeitgeist, are more readily accepted for publication. Once published, their findings, because they confirm the theory, are more often cited in theoretical articles. Has the theory been confirmed? Yes, but to an undecided extent. Is the theory in need of change? Yes, if only on the grounds that initial formulations are almost always in error. For a recent example, consider patients' reports of parental seduction and how they have changed with the advent of new knowledge about child abuse. Where are the data to support these reformulations? Almost unavailable because of the self-serving nature of the case study genre.

To put the point more strongly: there is no reason to believe, given the present case study tradition, that theory will *ever* change to any significant degree, or that it will be appreciably informed, refreshed, or amended by current clinical happenings. So long as Freud is seen as the prevailing authority, the clinical reports that become part of the literature will almost necessarily be in support of the received theory. We have seen how argument by authority tends to suppress polite disagreement and, by implication, the adversarial tradition. And so long as readers are not encouraged to differ with published reports, the evidential standing of these reports will be that much more inflated.

The missing element in all of this is a public forum. From its earliest beginnings, science—and empiricist science in particular—has prided itself on being fanatically democratic. Data belong to the public domain and are open to inspection or reanalysis by any interested party. Procedures are publicly available. Public procedures combined with public data make it possible for anyone with the proper training and apparatus to carry out standard experiments and thus determine whether a given finding can or cannot be replicated. "Old beliefs," writes Campbell, "are to be doubted until they have been reconfirmed by the methods of the new science. Persuasion is to be limited to egalitarian means, potentially accessible to all, that is, to visual and logical demonstrations (note how much of proof in Euclid is based on dependably shareable visual judgments)" (1986, p. 119).

As the new science developed, replication more and more became the road to persuasion, and replication depends to a very great extent on the model of participatory democracy. Campbell tells us that "a crucial part of the egalitarian, antiauthoritarian ideology of the seventeenth-century 'new science' was the ideal that each member of the scientific community could replicate a demonstration for himself . . . Each scientist was to be allowed to inspect the apparatus and try out the shared recipe." Restrict such open access and truth suffers: "A healthy community of truth seekers can flourish where such replication is possible. It becomes precarious where it is not" (p. 122).

Occult Practices

For an account of what may happen when these principles are not observed, we need look no further than the history of alchemy during the Renaissance. Although the distinction between alchemy and science is less sharp than popular stereotypes would suggest (see Vickers, 1984), there is no question but that alchemy relied heavily on secrecy and magic in clear violation of the egalitarian ethic of traditional science:

> The occult [of which alchemy was a part] has always been secretive, restricting knowledge to adepts or initiates, communicating only in hermetic forms or in messages designed to sabotage themselves (such as alchemical recipes in cipher or exotic foreign languages—Ethiopian, say—or with names of crucial substances or quantities omitted). Where scientific experiments are repeatable and public, occult experiments, or experiences, are personal and notoriously not repeatable (above all not in alchemy, where the absence of any established criteria for determining the purity or concentration of substances, solid or liquid, or of standardizing temperature, made for insuperable difficulties in emulation). (Vickers, 1984, pp. 41–42)

Once secrecy obtains a footing in the enterprise, it tends to elevate argument by authority and other more dubious (and diminishing) rhetorical figures over the careful sifting of the specimen of interest. As reductive rhetoric displaces evidence, we lose the ability to reach what Habermas (1971) has called an "uncompelled consensus" because the rich nature of the specimen is no longer available for all to examine. Reductive explanations of this kind were one of the unfortunate consequences of the conceptualist belief that only initiated observers could be fully sensitive to the full implications of the specimen, and even if their view was biased or incomplete, it still carried the day. Under these conditions, replication loses much of its leverage as a test of persuasion because failures of replication can be put down to poor technique, to an inexperienced or insensitive investigator, to lack of access to the proper ingredients, to a misreading of the recipe, or—in the last resort—to the principle that occult experiments are nonrepeatable. If that principle is scrupulously observed, then replication failure merely confirms the axiom and thus supports the general system. What Campbell calls "mutual monitoring" fails because procedures and data are no longer in the public domain.

Protected by its use of secrecy, arcane language, and reductive rhetoric from the challenges of the disbelievers, alchemy and the occult in general became even more fallible. It can be seen that this tradition had reached a dead end. As it grew more secret, it became even more of a closed system. "If a belief in numerology were abandoned, it would destroy the basis for alchemy and astrology; if a belief in astrology were abandoned, it would destroy alchemy, botanical medicine, and much else" (Vickers, 1984, p. 35). It could be argued that the closed system probably encouraged the need for secrecy and increased reliance on arcane ciphers and exotic languages, because any challenge would threaten the total web of belief, and thus every challenge was potentially destructive.

Not only was the occult system highly interdependent; its practitioners also maintained a protective attitude toward established theory. Truth was largely known and need only be embellished. In contrast to traditional science, practitioners of the occult

> never threw away anything, and much of the system elaborated in the Hellenistic period survives intact today. Modern astrology has absorbed some later planetary discoveries, and there are some sporadic instances of the application of quantitative techniques to mystical goals (as in Leonhard Thurneisser's use of quantitative analysis of urine to identify the three Paracelsian principles, mixing chemical

with analogical and metaphorical procedures), but by and large the occult sciences have gone on unchanged. (Vickers, 1984, p. 38)

As rhetoric became more diminished, appeals to authority replaced the full range of rhetorical figures. As procedures became exotic, self-destructive, or cabalistic, secrecy became the norm. To add to the disarray, words began taking over from things. As *reductive* rhetoric takes over from *descriptive* rhetoric, we see a clear change in the way alchemists approached language and the way in which they related language to the world. The contrast with empiricist science becomes increasingly sharpened:

In the [Galilean] scientific tradition . . . a clear distinction is made between words and things and between literal and metaphorical lan guage. The occult tradition does not recognize this distinction: Words are treated as if they are equivalent to things and can be substituted for them. Manipulate the one and you manipulate the other. Analogies, instead of being . . . explanatory devices subordinate to argument and proof, or heuristic tools to make models that can be tested, corrected, and abandoned if necessary, are, instead, modes of conceiving relationships in the universe that reify, rigidify, and ultimately come to dominate thought. (Vickers, 1984, p. 95)

A similar confusion surrounded other figures of speech. Whereas metaphor and simile were recognized by the new sciences as separate from the nonfigurative, normal level of discourse, quite a different position was taken by the occult sciences, which might mistake these same figures for representations of reality. The metaphor was treated as equivalent to the object it represented; comparison was collapsed into identity. What was even more destructive to clear thinking, the use of a given metaphor was not seen as a provisional means of representing a particular happening but as representing its very essence. This form of concrete thinking contributed to the reluctance to change, noted above, and to a belief in words as talismans: "The word is not merely like a quality of the thing it designates, such as its color or weight; it is, or exactly represents, its essence or substance" (Walker, 1958; quoted in Vickers, 1984, p. 119). Robert Boyle had earlier attacked the language of the occult tradition for its "obscure, ambiguous . . . aenigmatical way of expressing what they pretend to teach . . . of playing with names at pleasure . . . so they will oftentimes give one thing many names" (quoted in Vickers, 1984, p. 114).

The fascination with empty rhetoric and the more magical features of language tended to draw attention away from the real world and back to the intricacies of the occult system. Less and less attention was paid to ways of validating the system or heeding exceptions to this or that rule. The system was sacred, to be preserved at all costs, and accessible only to those chosen few who understood its secret ways.

Psychoanalysis and Science

Psychoanalysis also prides itself on being a Galilean science and belonging to the mainstream of the scientific tradition. Freud was quite clear on this point. Grünbaum notes that "throughout his long career, Freud insisted that the psychoanalytic enterprise has the status of a natural [that is, empiricist] science. As he told us at the very end of his life, the explanatory gains from positing unconscious mental processes 'enabled psychology to take its place as a natural science like any other' " (Freud, 1933, p. 158; quoted in Grünbaum, 1984, p. 2). "The intellect and the mind [wrote Freud] are objects for scientific research in exactly the same way as any non-human things. Psychoanalysis has a special right to speak for the scientific *Weltanschauung*" (p. 159). In an earlier statement, Freud expressed his regret that the scientific standing of psychoanalysis was not obvious to others. "I have always felt it as a gross injustice that people have refused to treat psychoanalysis like any other science" (1925, p. 58).

Similar support comes from his followers: "Like every other scientist a psychoanalyst is an empiricist, who imaginatively infers functional and causal relations among his data" (Brenner, 1982, p. 5). Holt has described the profession as a "fledgling science" that is struggling to become respectable despite the fact that "it is hard to admit how little *proof* there is for any psychoanalytic hypothesis after all these years of use" (1984, p. 26).

These are brave words. At the same time, science is as science does. While it would like to be considered a paradigmatic empiricist science, certain aspects of psychoanalysis, as we have also seen, seem more occult than Galilean. As we have also seen, data are largely private and not accessible to the curious scholar who wants to see for himself and who, following the empiricist tradition, has every right to expect full disclosures. Part of this privacy is needed to protect the patient, but it has the effect of ruling out the traditional kinds of Baconian replication by participant-observation. This kind of secrecy not only becomes a rhetorical device in its own right, it leads directly to persuasion through an impoverished rhetoric that depends heavily on reductive explanation and on argument by authority.

Second, concern for the privacy of the patient leads to the dubious tradition of protection through disguise; thus, many of the details of so-called case reports are actually falsified, but the line where truth stops and disguise begins is never made clear, and as a result, the vast majority of case reports have little or no archival value. With almost any case presentation, we can raise the classic alchemist's challenge: Is the author being *grudging* or *generous*? Should the text be read as a complete and open description of the clinical happening or should we consider him grudging, bound by secrecy, hedging his facts with both revealed and concealed forms of disguise and therefore not to be taken at face value?

Third, there is no precedent in the psychoanalytic literature for the kind of open discussion of conflicting findings that is central to the Galilean scientific tradition. Negative instances are almost never published and unsuccessful cases, as we have seen, are practically never reported.

Further inspection of the case study genre reveals some additional parallels with the occult tradition. There is, first of all, an overriding reliance on empty metaphor and a tendency to substitute word for thing (see Spence, 1982, 1987). The use of this type of (reductive) metaphor interferes with careful observation, because the true nature of the referent is always falsified by its name. As we have seen in Chapter 4, metaphor tends to be used in a highly concrete and dogmatic manner; it does not represent a provisional or tentative means of representing the world but, rather, is accepted as a final statement. Second, as I noted earlier, there is the temptation to use secrecy as a metaphor and to rely wherever possible on the rhetorical figure of metalepsis, calling on causative agents from the past to account for present effects. These agents can never be made visible and thus examined directly. We might consider, in this connection, the role of infantile wishes in dream formation: they are treated as real objects, but they operate largely as metaphors for the unseen. Third, critical dialogue is handicapped by the theory-laden nature of many of the facts. Only verbatim samples of clinical happenings make it possible for an outside observer to determine how much of a given statement is observation and how much theory, but because of the scarcity of clinical data in the public domain, this recourse is essentially ruled out. The specimen, in other words, is never fully explored.

Rather than exploit the full resources of conceptualist science and make full use of all available rhetorical figures in an effort to explore, as fully as possible, the complexity of the specimen, psychoanalysis has opted for a reduced conceptualism that slights the specimen, skimps on the detail, and models itself on the harder sciences. Rather than recognize the ambiguity of the clinical material and the extent to which meaning is a projection of the analyst, current case reports treat reality in a largely positivistic and objective fashion. Covering laws are invoked prematurely, giving the impression that more is known than is actually the case.

What further similarities with the alchemists can we discover? Truth is taken as largely discovered, standard beliefs are to be accepted rather than doubted, and the old is given preference over the new. Psychoanalysis is traditionally reluctant to consider new alternatives and revise its theories and models.

Since the critical findings are largely outside the public domain, traditional forms of replication are ruled out and persuasion relies largely on appeal to authority, secrecy, and the extended use of an impoverished rhetoric. Where the earlier investigator, schooled in the classical trivium of logic, grammar, and rhetoric, could choose from among more than two hundred tropes to describe his specimen, the current investigator has access to little more than enargia, metaphor, metalepsis, and metonomy. As a result, the specimen can never be described with the detail it deserves, and it could be argued that not since Freud's five cases have we had the kind of rich description that is presupposed by the Aristotelian tradition.

A Specimen Case

To explore the use of an impoverished and reductive rhetoric in the standard psychoanalytic case, it seems useful at this point to take a detailed look at a recent clinical report and examine the form of the argument, the use of different kinds of rhetorical figures, and the interplay of Aristotelian, occult, and Galilean forms of reasoning in the service of both description and persuasion. Such an analysis should highlight the different kinds of rhetorical influence the author of a case study can bring to bear on the reader and make clear just how these (largely reductive) tools of persuasion compare with the more traditional figures.

As my target article I have selected a case report of a childhood seduction and its subsequent effects on the victim. The paper is entitled "Reconstruction of an Early Seduction and Its Aftereffects" (Williams, 1987). We can identify at least two domains of discourse: On the one hand, there is a series of events in real life concerning a real patient, his upbringing, his memory of this upbringing, and the use made of these memories in two specific periods of psychoanalysis with two different analysts. The two treatments brought about two quite different outcomes, and this difference becomes one of the points at issue. On the other hand, there are also the thoughts and comments of the author *about* the first domain of discourse. The two parts do not always agree: the author/analyst sometimes makes statements that either do not correspond to the details of the patient's experience or raise the suggestion that she was not sufficiently curious about gaps or inconsistencies in the original record. We are reminded of the role of Lambert Strether, the narrator in Henry James's *The Ambassadors*, who is forever getting in the way of a clear view of the events and filtering what takes place through *his* eyes, the eyes of a visiting American, set in his ways, who uses too much imagination in some respects and too little in others.

Of equal importance to the two domains of discourse I have already described is another voice—Freud's—which is quoted early in the article and which forms a subtext for much of the argument. Because of its importance to the overall argument, this passage deserves to be quoted in full. Freud is describing the nature of reconstruction:

> Scenes . . . which date from such an early period . . . and which further lay claim to such an extraordinary significance for the history of the case, are as a rule not reproduced as recollections, but have to be divined—constructed—gradually and laboriously from an aggregate of indications . . . It seems to me absolutely equivalent to recollection, if the memories are replaced (as in the present case) by dreams the analysis of which invariably leads back to the same scene and which reproduce every portion of its content in an inexhaustible variety of new shapes. Indeed, dreaming is another kind of remembering, though one that is subject to the conditions that rule at night and to the laws of dream formation. It is this recurrence in dreams

that I regard as the explanation of the fact that the patients themselves gradually acquire a profound conviction of the reality of these
primal scenes, a conviction which is in no respect inferior to one
based on recollection. (pp. 146–147)

This statement by the founder of psychoanalysis is clearly intended as
an epigraph for the paper. We are being prepared for some kind of
validation or corroboration of its main thesis. We are led to believe
that 1) dreams are lawful; 2) dreams are equivalent to memories; and
3) conviction in the dreamer can be used as a form of validation.

Further inspection of the topic paragraph also provides some insight
into the rhetorical subtext of the target article. It is clear from the
outset that the author has no intention of quarreling with any part of
Freud's argument; his authority will go unchallenged throughout. But
if these assertions are allowed to stand, the reader begins to feel
increasingly pessimistic about the clarity or precision of the author's
reasoning and about her ability to draw her own conclusions from the
specimen, independent of the teachings of standard theory. If her findings did not, in fact, support these teachings, what would be their fate?
Not only was she incurious about the clinical details, but she has
become Freud's alter ego, protective of his point of view and probably
not open to disconfirming or embarrassing evidence.

Turning to the target article, we find that the early childhood of the
patient quickly becomes the focus of the discussion. When he was two,
his parents were divorced and "immediately following the divorce, the
mother left on an extended trip that in some family versions lasted ten
months, but according to her only five. The patient was left in the care
of an elderly aunt and uncle, who in turn entrusted the boy to the care
of a strict nurse and [Joseph], a friendly male servant to whom,
according to the patient and family members, the boy was very
attached" (pp. 147–148). The author then turns to the patient's later
development in childhood and adolescence and describes his adult
adjustment difficulties and his search for relief through psychoanalysis. The first analysis was broken off after some eight years of dis-
continuous treatment at a time when the patient felt he had made no
progress; he was referred to the author for a second analysis. During
the course of the first treatment, there were multiple indications that
some childhood trauma had taken place, but the details of the event
were neither fully reconstructed nor forcefully addressed.

We have now reached the heart of the argument. The author suggests that failure to focus attention on the seduction was responsible for lack of success in the first treatment and that when it became the center of the clinical work (as it did in the second analysis), the patient's symptoms began to diminish and he reached a successful resolution of his problems. But to make this argument, the author must provide convincing evidence that a seduction had actually taken place, and here is where the paper becomes its most unsatisfactory. We are given no direct evidence that the early seduction (by the male servant) had actually taken place; instead, we are given only *summaries* (not verbatim reports) of repetitive dreams about ugly buildings, overflowing toilets, floating feces, and a bedroom with many beds. Despite the importance of this material to the argument, no single dream is ever reported in its entirety. We are also told by the patient, after the reconstruction was made, that he remembers going to the servant's home—not once, but many times—and that relatives had told him how attached he was to the servant and how he followed him around. But such memories, together with the repetitive dreams, are merely *consistent* with a possible seduction; they add nothing to its proof. Once again, we are troubled by the author's failure to raise this distinction and show us a skeptical mind at work.

But something else is going on as well. Not only is the seduction hypothesis never examined in a critical manner, but over the course of the paper its status changes from hypothesis to fact. On page 152 we are told once again about the male servant who, "as the first analysis revealed and the second analysis confirmed [sic], had molested his young charge. In a clinical presentation in a circle of analysts, the first analyst reported he had come to this conclusion from a few screen memories and repetitive dreams of the patient; he saw this molestation as a homosexual trauma; it apparently was not pursued further." In the next paragraph, the author describes how she told the patient that she *suspected* that he had been seduced and molested by the male servant, based on the evidence of the repetitive dreams (and also influenced, we may assume, by the conviction of the first analyst). But suspicion quickly changes to conviction. On the next page, we are told of the "seduction by Joseph" (no qualification); further references to "the seduction" occur repeatedly throughout the article, in the title, and in the abstract. The author (and evidently the patient) is convinced of its factual basis, and in the next-to-last paragraph, we are told that "the seduction [now a simple fact] hindered his freedom to develop normally; he lived in shackles until he learned to remove them" (p. 163).

In a general way, the possibility of early seduction by the male servant at a time when the father had left the home, the mother was away on an extended trip, and the patient was left in the care of elderly relatives seems a plausible hypothesis that *could* explain the repetitive dreams, the patient's fear of closeness, and other aspects of his symptom picture. It ranks as a *possible* but not a *necessary* cause of the clinical details. But the distinction between the two kinds of cause is not examined in any depth. These questions are all the more relevant because of the ambiguity of the evidence. Here is another case where interpretation seems to masquerade as explanation, an interpretation that receives no particular sanction beyond the fact that it agrees with standard theory.

What more is needed in the way of confirming evidence? Or, to ask a more Aristotelian question, what else could a qualified observer discover in this specimen and how could his findings be presented in a manner that would persuade the reader that he had reached the bottom of its complexity? First, we would expect to find clarification of the memory as its significance was unfolded in the course of the analysis. Additional details might also be recovered, even at an early stage, which would make the remembered event more clearly a first-person experience that happened to the patient and was remembered by him. No such additional facts are reported. The patient recovers a memory of going home with Joseph not once "but many times," but nothing more emerges in the way of new memories or dreams. The dilapidated buildings in the repetitive dreams are taken to be references to Joseph's home, but their form does not seem to change after the reconstruction is made explicit. Thus the hypothesis of early seduction has about the same evidential standing at the end of treatment as it did at the beginning, but it is treated as if confirmed by the clinical data and, by the end of the article, confirmed beyond question. To the author's satisfaction, perhaps, but not to the reader's.

Whatever his discomfort, the captive reader has no way of entering into a discussion with either the author or the findings (here is where the lack of public data becomes especially telling). The target article brings into focus some of the standard problems of current reporting—its reliance on an impoverished narrative and on a highly reductive rhetoric that tends to substitute conclusions for facts.

Reading Williams, one never has the feeling that she is allowing herself to "surrender" (in Ricoeur's phrase) to the full range of meanings that might be found in the specimen, either admitting that the story still puzzled her in places, or wrestling with her discoveries and making a more resolute attempt to capture them in language. Whenever the choice lies between grounding her explanation in a covering law (that is, infantile seduction) and a contingent, one-of-a-kind happening, the author always chooses the former. But giving her account the stamp of Galilean science does not necessarily convince the reader, and as I have argued in Chapter 3, to frame explanations in covering laws tends to leave out the most important aspect of the clinical happening.

Writing in this genre—halfway between a full-blooded rhetorical account and a more abstract and scientific description—effectively prevents the skeptical reader from making contact with the clinical material, from reaching his own conclusions from the evidence, and from applying his therapeutic expertise to the material in question. More specifically, it prevents the analyst/reader from applying his "analyzing instrument" to the full extent of its capacity.

Perhaps if the narrative had been more persuasive, the reader would be less impatient. Freud was ruefully aware of the similarity between his case reports and narrative fiction, and in the hands of a master storyteller, the standard genre is highly effective. But if the craft is imperfectly practiced, if the narrative smoothing is perhaps too obvious, or if hypothesis slides too quickly into explanation, then we are left feeling dissatisfied and unpersuaded. Rather than suspend whatever disbelief we may bring to the account at the outset, we tend to double our skepticism with each unsupported assertion. In the final reckoning, bad case reports read like bad fiction; they leave us feeling unhappy and argued with—certainly not convinced or informed.

But of course, the case report is not only bad fiction. It presents itself—particularly when written in the current empiricist spirit—as a piece of the truth, a sample of clinical reporting that has a permanent bearing on psychoanalytic theory. The wording of the title, "Reconstruction of an Early Seduction and Its Aftereffects," sounds definitive and final, and does not convey any of the underlying ambiguities that appear in the case report. An uncritical reading of the target article would seem to support the standard assumption that early seduction can have significant effects on later development, that derivatives of this seduction can be detected in dreams many years later, that dreams do indeed behave like memories and that early experiences are law-fully transformed into dream content, and that the proper reconstruction of an early event can significantly affect the course of psycho-analysis. A simple reading of the title or an uncritical reading of the article would suggest that Freud's formulation was essentially correct and that his hypothesis stands confirmed in all its details—a truly remarkable state of affairs. A more critical reading suggests something quite different. Not only is standard theory *not* being confirmed, but the specimen is being examined in a largely uncritical fashion. Of particular interest is the relation between the quotation from Freud on the traumatizing effects of early experience and the clinical findings reported in the case study. The statement by Freud gives permission, as it were, to look for the long-term effects of early trauma in later dreams and associations. The statement by the first analyst that he had found evidence for early trauma further reinforces Freud's argument and further prepares the way for its confirmation. Against this background, any evidence that is consistent with the formulation tends to be judged sufficient.

The difference in our response to the clinical findings underlines the obvious fact that meanings in the first domain of discourse—the patient's life—are far from transparent. They are always being colored by the context of events and the author's theoretical assumptions. The theory-laden nature of the facts poses a particular problem for this kind of account because the standard narrative method may simply be unequipped to present the story along with its context of understanding. We can put the point more directly by saying that the standard narrative approach disarms the reader into believing that a simple story is being told—but this is clearly not the case. Seen in that light, we can think of the standard case study method as serving a specific kind of rhetorical function that is designed to tempt the reader into a suspension of disbelief. He is persuaded to put himself into the hands of the author, as opposed to having a conversation with the author about the merits of the argument.

An Alternative Reading

In contrast to the rather superficial narrative approach taken by the author, we might consider how a conceptualist scientist would look at this specimen. First, he would assume that not everything important is visible on first reading, so it follows that he must allow himself to be drawn deeper into the clinical material and begin to explicate the latent meanings. Keeping in mind the many ways in which meanings can be transformed, we can consider this piece of clinical material taken from early in the analysis:

> In a related series of repetitive dreams, the patient comes to some dirty and ugly buildings. He goes in and enters a bedroom with many beds. Some are occupied. The patient finds himself in bed, and a man joins him, lying against his back. The man does something to the patient's anus, producing great anxiety in him, both within the dream and as [the patient] recounted it. (Williams, 1987, p. 150)

A rhetorical analysis might begin by paying attention to the original wording used by the patient and to the ways in which the significant content was first expressed. When we are told that the man "does something to the patient's anus" that causes anxiety both within the dream and within the hour (as it was recounted), is there perhaps a link between the three locations   *within* the anus, *within* the dream, and *within* the hour? Does the man lying against his back represent the analyst who sits behind him during the session with an agenda of repeated attempts to reconstruct the infantile seduction? Could it be that the analyst's repeated attempts to interpret the infantile seduction were themselves experienced as a kind of anal penetration, originating as they do behind the patient (who was lying on the couch) and combining both anxious and pleasurable elements? Williams tells us that "analysis itself was for this patient like a seduction which he tried to prevent by keeping his distance and reserve . . ." (pp. 155–156); could we be even more specific and treat the repeated reconstructions as a series of anal stimulations?

As the analysis continues and interpretations accumulate,

> more material from this traumatic past was recovered. One such notable experience surfaced in the following dream. A man who is lying down on a bed is lifting up a little boy whom he holds suspended horizontally above himself. As the boy looks down he sees a large erect penis. As the patient depicted this scene, he shuddered with disgust. Mr. B. felt he had been able to dream and relate this dream only because he trusted me more. (p. 154)

The author treats this material as an expression of further memories about the seduction and thus as confirmation of the truth about the reconstruction. But the Aristotelian scientist, in his efforts to track down the disguised meaning of the specimen, might take quite a different approach. Could the man lying on the bed and lifting the little boy represent the analyst, who is supporting and stimulating the regressed patient? Does the erect penis, viewed from above, express the patient's awesome impression of the analyst's all-powerful and never-tiring store of wisdom, the source of repeated and unsettling interpretations?

The choice of rhetorical figure clearly affects our reading of the clinical specimen. If we begin with the familiar figure of metalepsis, we look for distant causes of present events and treat the cited dream as the present result of something that happened long ago. Infantile seduction by Joseph is now represented (and, it should be noted, with minimal transformation) by the image of the man lying on a bed and holding a small boy up in the air. An interpretation along these lines is reinforced by the use of a second figure—enargia—which tempts us to treat the details as pictorial, concrete, and essentially untransformed. But if we start with the rhetorical figure of *syllepsis,* then we are on the lookout for ways in which the meanings may change, depending on context and tone. According to this reading, the controlling figure on the bed is the analyst, not Joseph; the small boy is the patient who is in the analyst's care and dependent on his support; and the erect penis is the source of repeated "penetrating" interpretations that are viewed with a combination of trust and disgust. If we are on the lookout for word play and for ways in which one meaning may slide into another, then we are necessarily on guard against a literal reading of the dream and view metalepsis with suspicion, seeing it as a rhetorical figure in the service of received theory. If we minimize metalepsis, we may also be less tempted to emphasize *enargia* as the second controlling figure. I would note that the choice of figure determines the meaning of the specimen, just as, during the Middle Ages, the choice of similitude governed interpretation. I would also note that the choice of one figure can easily blind us to another. Because the analyst seems intent on proving that some kind of seduction took place at an early age (a position that implicitly endorses metalepsis), she tends to view all the clinical material as evidence for this thesis. This line of argument reinforces the use of enargia; she is unwittingly committing the error of misplaced concreteness. As the details are taken more and more literally, she is less able to consider the possibility of word play and the use of syllepsis.

Reconstruction or Metalepsis?

It seems clear that the clinical material cited by Williams does not necessarily lead to one and only one interpretation. Arguments can be found to support the thesis that the patient had been anally seduced at a young age, but such an interpretation depends heavily on the use of two rhetorical figures: enargia, to highlight the specific details in the clinical material, and metalepsis, to point to causal influences from the past. The conclusion, therefore, is significantly influenced by these rhetorical choices; it does not flow inevitably from the clinical specimen. We begin to realize that Williams's decision to see the material in this manner presupposes the use of enargia and metalepsis as organizing principles. Choose other figures and other meanings come to light. Once we realize that psychoanalysis speaks with a rhetorical voice, we can begin to search for particular rhetorical figures. Once we lose sight of our Aristotelian heritage, however, and believe that we are working in a Galilean tradition, we lose track of the different rhetorical possibilities and begin to believe that a particular reading is the only reading and that it derives necessarily and inevitably from the target specimen.

How well does this particular clinical report stand up as an example of Galilean science? We quote once again from Campbell:

> The ideology of science was and is explicitly antiauthoritarian, antitraditional, antirevelational, and individualistic. Truth is yet to be revealed ... The community of scientists is to stay together in focused disputation, monitoring and keeping each other honest until some working consensus emerges (but conformity of belief per se is rejected as an acceptable goal). (Campbell, 1986, p. 119)

We are immediately struck by a number of vivid contrasts between these assumptions and those made by the author of the target article. As we have seen, Williams takes Freud's original assertion about the function of early memories as the subtext of her presentation and honors this old belief rather than questions it. Truth, she seems to assume, is already known and needs only to be reconfirmed; the details are unlikely to change. As we have also seen, persuasion is far from a democratic procedure because the facts surrounding the presumed infantile seduction are incompletely presented; they are certainly not "potentially accessible" to all interested parties. What is more, persuasion tends to be arbitrary and authoritarian and depends heavily on the prior statements of Freud and other expert witnesses (especially the first analyst). Because the relevant data are not made public, there is no opportunity for open discussion of alternative meanings of the evidence, a dialogue that would lead to the "uncompelled consensus" recommended by Habermas. On the contrary, the conclusion is explicitly compelled and as a result quite unsurprising—and rather unconvincing.

These contrasts come to light because Williams is working within neither an Aristotelian nor a Galilean tradition. While she appears to be presenting us with a documented reconstruction that supports one of Freud's "covering laws," we have instead a reading of the specimen that arbitrarily relies on two rhetorical figures to make its point. But because its Aristotelian grounding is never made explicit, we are deceived into treating the case report as a piece of contemporary science.

We now see the dangers of this compromised genre, which aspires to normal science before its time. Conclusions are emphasized over evidence, one interpretation is stressed over a range of alternatives, and the specific detail of the specimen is exchanged for the colorless language of a scientific report. In the attempt to be objective, Williams has omitted the specific words the patient used to describe his initial fears, his changing memories of the childhood incident, his dreams, and his reactions to the analyst's reconstructive interpretations. Sampling this language would allow us to get closer to the analyzed patient as he was experiencing the transference and give us a way of sampling the ambience of the treatment. Given the patient's specific utterances, we would be able to apply a range of rhetorical figures to their understanding and, in this way, come to discover much more about the treatment process. Deprived of his language, however, we are also deprived of our favorite figures, because they can only be applied to the concrete terms. When the patient's speech is paraphrased, we are helpless to discover further rhetorical shadings. When the analyst's speech is concealed, we learn next to nothing about the countertransference.

Screening the reader from the here-and-now utterances of patient and analyst tends to leave him out of the "conversation" and make him almost completely dependent on the judgment and wisdom of the author. But as we have seen, the meaning of a clinical specimen is almost never transparent; thus it is all the more necessary that we do not fall back on authoritarian forms of argument. To depend on a single opinion is perilous enough in the average situation; to depend on it when meanings are frequently ambiguous, context-determined, and open to this or that rhetorical analysis is to confound the problem all the more.

This compromised genre—single-case analysis masquerading as Galilean science—has a further dangerous consequence. As psychoanalysis tries to become more "scientific," it may well lose its Aristotelian heritage along the way and, in the long run, belong to neither tradition. Will it suffer the same fate as alchemy and the other occult sciences? We are reminded uncomfortably of the alchemists, with their faith in closed theory, which sees no need for change, and with their suspicion of full disclosure, because for them, secrecy was power.

III

Implications

7 Happy Examples and Alternative Formulations

When Freud abandoned his inductive training around the turn of the century and chose instead to present illustrative examples only, he left a mark on the form and content of clinical reporting that is still visible today. Even though he was indicating a personal preference in his style of investigation as much as discarding the Galilean approach, subsequent investigators seem to think that Freud's anecdotal approach, with its focus on convenient examples, is the only way to do clinical science and that any attempt to follow traditional, Galilean procedures would violate a sacred trust. If we pick up any issue of the *Journal of the American Psychoanalytic Association* we find a friendly defense of received theory buttressed by one or more supporting anecdotes and quotations from like-minded authorities. Current case reports are illustrative but incomplete. Because complete clinical reports are never presented, critical data are frequently withheld from the public domain, making it impossible for an outside reader to examine systematically either the methods of current practice or the extent to which current practice supports contemporary theory. The general erosion in clinical reporting since Freud's original five cases is not only disturbing in its own right, it also casts an ominous light on the standing of psychoanalytic theory, because if current documentation is as meager as it seems, how do we know that theory has anything significant to say about practice?

The fact that in the almost one hundred years since the Dora case was written we have been given no better documentation of the central psychoanalytic assumptions than we find in the original five cases also raises a question about the function of current case reports. Rather than debate the covering laws of received theory and test them against a wide range of clinical observations, the typical report plays a more reassuring role, paying lip service to the general assumptions underlying psychoanalysis and carrying the message to the doubtful reader that there are other practitioners who also believe what he believes and practice as he practices. The message is implicit in any number of clinical accounts, but because it is largely rhetorical, it does not need to be supported by data. Since the published reports tend to confirm received theory, they lend credence to the belief that the official wisdom is largely correct and in no danger of being upset by new findings.

When clinical observations are used to support received theory, as we have seen in Chapter 6, they are used to illustrate and persuade rather than to discover. Language is used to determine a point of view and establish a set of conclusions rather than as a means of representing the world. If we are interested in the latter question, we would call attention to the ways in which the accounts of the analytic process in Williams's paper were incomplete and ambiguous, to the many questions that still remain unanswered about the patient's past, and to the lack of convincing evidence to support the thesis that the interpretation of infantile incest played an important role in the patient's later development. If we are interested in the role of language as representation, we would also raise questions about the metaphoric nature of much of our theory and call attention to the ways in which our favorite terms conceal as much as they disclose. Finally, we would focus on the fact that the metaphoric nature of many of our concepts makes it difficult, if not impossible, to either confirm or disconfirm them, thus putting into question the general relation between theory and evidence.

A superficial analysis of the current literature makes it appear that psychoanalysis is a science like any other, dependent on new evidence to bring theory into contact with practice. But a closer look at the actual case studies and theoretical discussions shows that in contrast to normal science, the evidence in psychoanalysis is largely anecdotal and incomplete and is almost never used to disconfirm established beliefs. Thus the professional literature serves a largely rhetorical function that is designed for reassurance, but closer examination reveals many gaps in the underlying reasoning and a tendency to persuade the reader more through illustration than documentation. Once again, we see how we have exchanged a Galilean, inductive tradition that pre-

sents a series of cases from which the reader can draw his own conclusions for an Aristotelian tradition that presents examples of the
general rule and depends on the appeal of the specimen to carry the
argument. But it is a watered-down conceptualism that omits the
telling detail of "thick description."

Presentation of a single example would, in many cases, be sufficient
if it were truly a representative instance of a larger class of cases. Under
such conditions, the careful analysis and discussion of the specimen
can be a useful method of exposition. But if the example is atypical
or too casually described, then we are in no position to draw general
conclusions from its characteristics, and any attempt to base an argument on it becomes more a piece of rhetoric than a branch of science.
It misleads more than it clarifies.

Yet despite the evidential flaws of current case reports, no one com-
plains. There are no letters to current journals calling attention to this
or that logical fallacy, to the lack of a public data base, or to the
pernicious effects of concealment and disguise. It can be argued that
we have a tolerance for shoddy reporting because we were persuaded
by Freud that his case histories were necessarily incomplete, that their
fragmented form was unavoidable, given the nature of the material
and the difficulty of reporting the many levels of evidence, and was
thus dictated by the nature of the material. By way of justification, he
argued that complete reports would compromise the identity of the
patient (1905) and disguised reports would compromise the integrity
of the communication (1909; both references in Sulloway, 1991).

But as we have seen, Freud also argued that "it is very remarkable
how the whole task becomes impossible if a reservation is allowed at
any single place" (1913, p. 136n). This statement, used to explain why
no concessions to the Basic Rule were to be allowed in beginning a
psychoanalysis, can also apply to the need to present a complete and
uncensored account of the clinical happening. It can serve as a scientific Bill of Rights for the clinical investigator. So long as we give
permission to our colleagues to tell less than the full story, we have
reneged on our role as scientists. The need to protect the patient can
be used to withhold any number of embarrassing revelations about
any number of issues having nothing to do with the patient; in the
final accounting, incomplete and anecdotal reporting in the service of
protecting the doctor-patient relationship can be used to conceal a
basic defect in the theory and delay for months or even years necessary

changes in technique. It goes without saying that incomplete reporting can also be employed in the service of concealing mistakes and preventing others from being witness to our blundering attempts to frame an interpretation when the words fail to come out as planned, from forgetting an obvious reference and suffering an embarrassing correction, or from any number of other common mistakes that we would rather forget than reveal.

We would seem to enjoy our present anecdotal, unsystematic form of presentation not only because Freud suggested it in the first place, but for precisely the same reasons Freud's patient from the Austrian government enjoyed the right to conceal secrets whenever he wished: it allows everyone the freedom to practice as he wishes, with no need to justify his response. But the price we pay for this freedom is a theory that is gradually losing touch with clinical practice and a set of clinical happenings that, because they are unreported, are never adequately understood.

Perils of Incomplete Reporting

A moment's thought will show that once a tradition of incomplete reporting has been established, it can be used to justify any theory. When only positive instances of a covering law are selected for publication, the reader has no way of knowing how many times a happy instance occurs naturally, how many times the law has been disconfirmed, or what is the proportion of positive to negative instances of instantiation. From the millions of clinical observations made since the beginning of psychoanalysis, it is obviously possible to pick out a sizable number that will confirm the central assumptions of whatever theory happens to be in fashion. So long as the clinical literature follows the tradition of incomplete reporting, we have no guarantee that the majority (perhaps even the totality) of published observations have not been selected for the single purpose of supporting established theory.

In his now-famous critique of medical education written just after the turn of the century, Flexner devoted a scathing chapter to the defects of "sectarian" medicine—allopathy, homeopathy, osteopathy, and so on: "The sectarian," he argued, "begins with his mind made up. He possesses in advance a general formula, which the particular instance is going to illustrate, verify, reaffirm, even though he may not know just how. One may be sure that facts so read will make good what is expected of them; that only that will be seen which will sustain its expected function; that every appeal noted will be dutifully loyal to the revelation in which favor the observer is predisposed; the human mind is so constituted" (1910, pp. 156–157).

The moral is clear—"the way to be unscientific is to be partial" (p. 92)—and the same teaching applies today. Not only are negative instances almost never reported, but the reader is never told the size of the full sample under consideration. If we assume that there are some three thousand analysts currently practicing in this country and that each of them is treating five cases, then a series of five reports showing a link, let us say, between unanalyzable symptoms and an early history of child abuse would not be very telling; this number represents only .03 percent of all possible cases (five out of fifteen thousand). Without a clear understanding of the size of the total sample from which these observations are drawn, the report of a small series of incidents, no matter how intriguing or provocative, is essentially meaningless.

In a recent paper by Waugaman on patients' use of first names, we are told in the opening sentence that "it is rare for a patient in analysis to speak of his parents by their first name." In the next paragraph, we are told that "using the parent's first name unconsciously signifies an oedipal transgression—it constitutes doing what one's other parent but not oneself is permitted to do" (1990, pp. 167, 168). Grounds for the first sentence are never given, and since the author provides no reason to believe that he has sampled the phenomenon in a systematic manner, we have no reason to accept his statement as true. Grounds for the second statement are suggested in the course of the paper, but these data stem almost entirely from a sample of five patients, and once again, we realize that a small set of positive instances is not sufficient to generate a lawful conclusion. When do patients violate the rule and use first names? in what proportion of all analyzed cases? In what proportion of these cases does it represent an oedipal transgression? In what proportion is this behavior caused by some other factor? We simply do not know, and the author seems uninterested in providing background information.

The argument is further weakened by the fact that no special precautions were taken to keep track of *all* uses of first names, and it seems doubtful whether the ordinary kind of process notes can be relied upon to maintain an exhaustive record of this kind. Without such a record, the reported findings—largely anecdotal—and the various conclusions are largely meaningless. But if, for example, the author had been able to make tape recordings of his five cases, enter the transcripts into a computer, and carry out a systematic search for parents' first names using one of the commercial software packages now available, the findings would stand on a much firmer foundation. Even the small size of the sample (N = 5) would matter much less if the record keeping had been reliable and exhaustive. As it stands, Waugaman's paper is merely another anecdotal study, mildly informative but not definitive, and not a contribution to a secure and accumulating knowledge base.

The tradition of incomplete reporting, carrying with it an implicit focus on the positive instance as a way of proving the general law, bears an obvious affinity to the Aristotelian tradition and speaks to a conception of science that existed in the days before the Newtonian revolution. But as we have seen, everything depends on the extent to which the instance represents the larger class. A true Aristotelian would first make sure that his specimen was representative; under these conditions, his elaboration of its particularities would provide useful information. But as this tradition is applied in current clinical reporting, an author merely pretends that his specimens are representative, and because they usually are not, his conclusions are largely fallacious.

This concentration on the happy example also speaks to another tradition that has an important connection with Freudian politics. From the very start of the psychoanalytic movement, Freud was determined to see that the clinical findings supported *his* theory and not those of Adler or Jung or another outsider. Adler was dismissed not because his observations were unlikely but because his theory was wrong; it verged on the incomprehensible. He used the wrong terms— he spoke of "masculine protest" when he should have been speaking of "repression"—and he neglected the importance of the unconscious and of sexuality (Gay, 1988, pp. 221–222). In a letter to Jung on June 18, 1909, Freud described Adler as astute and original but "not oriented to the psychological; he aims past it to the biological" (cited in Gay, 1988, pp. 220–221). After their relationship worsened and Adler was expelled from the Vienna Psychoanalytic Society, Freud told Jones in a letter of August 9, 1911: "as for the internal dissension with Adler, it was likely to come and I have ripened the crisis. It is the revolt of an abnormal individual driven mad by ambition, his influence on others depending on his strong terrorism and sadismus" (cited in Gay, 1988, p. 223).

Similar polemics were directed at Jung when he began to question the role of sexuality and some of the other central assumptions of the theory. Freud found him similar to Adler ("it is the same mechanism and the identical reaction as in Adler's case"—letter to Jones, December 26, 1912; cited in Gay, 1988, p. 235). As their differences increased, Freud wrote Ferenczi that "we must expect wicked things from Jung . . . Everything that strays from our truths has official applause on its side. It is quite possible that this time they will really bury us after they have so often sung us the dirge in vain. . . . [This] will change much in our fate, but nothing in that of science. We are in possession of the truth; I am as certain as I was fifteen years ago" (letter of May 8, 1913; cited in Gay, 1988, p. 237). We read the last sentence with a sinking feeling, for what could make it more apparent that established truths are far superior to new findings?

Conspicuously missing in these debates is any discussion of the clinical observations that might support Freud against Adler, or Jung against Freud. We get the strong impression that established theory—the theory of Freud's papers collected in the *Standard Edition*—is sacred and that facts are expendable. Adler was wrong because of his way of looking at the data; his approach was too biological, and thus his standing as a psychoanalyst suspect. Jung would seem to be largely right in his assessment many years later: "I criticize in Freudian psychology a certain narrowness and bias, and, in 'Freudians,' a certain unfree, sectarian spirit of intolerance and fanaticism" (letter to J. H. van der Hoop, January 14, 1946; cited in Gay, 1988, p. 238). In the debate with Jung, clinical observations once again took second place to accepted theory, and Jung was criticized "for being gullible about occult phenomena, and infatuated with oriental religion; [Freud] viewed with sardonic and unmitigated skepticism Jung's defense of religious feelings as an integral element in mental health" (Gay, 1988, p. 238).

If theory is sacred and more important than clinical observation, then we begin to understand more precisely why psychoanalysts came to accept a tradition of incomplete reporting and a focus on the positive instance. Clinical findings are used largely to support received theory; they function as examples that instantiate a covering law. If a certain brand of theory is to be reinforced and perpetuated, there is no need to report all observations. Only positive instances are needed, and it is always possible, as we have seen, to find one confirming case. The collection of data in our clinical records thus plays a rhetorical, not an archival function.

It goes without saying that there is a critical difference between a data base that supplies an occasional positive instance to be used as a clarifying example of a covering law and a data base that includes both positive and negative instances in the same proportion as they occur in the real world and therefore allows a systematic testing of fruitful hypotheses. Psychoanalysis, to date, still has no data base in the second sense of the term.

Public and Private Uses of Evidence

This fascination with the positive instance cannot be entirely attributed to an outdated Aristotelian tradition. We must also consider the way in which public reporting is inadvertently contaminated by more clinical and therapeutic considerations. In his role as a scientist presenting evidence for a pending hypothesis, the author-analyst finds it difficult to abandon totally his role as clinician accustomed to making interpretations to his patient on evidence that is sometimes less than ideal. Unfortunately, the rules that work in one arena do not always apply in the other, and it would seem that much of the bad logic in clinical reporting can be attributed to this confusion of roles.

In this vein, we might consider the following clinical vignette from Ramzy (1974). Some time before the hour in question, the analyst announced that he would be taking a two-week vacation. The week before the vacation was to begin, the patient began the hour as follows:

> Well, before I came up here I went back home since I forgot to leave a cheque with my cleaning lady. Well, she wasn't around and when I was driving up here I was kind of worried. She is sort of an old lady, maybe in her late 50's or early 60's. Maybe she's sick or some such. So I was telling myself while I was driving up here I better go and call some friend of mine and see what happened to her. And immediately it also struck me that: 'Well, what if she is really sick and can't work?' That would be kind of horrible. In Kansas a

cleaning lady is not so easy to find, especially the one that you don't have to tell her what to do and she will just automatically do . . . It was pretty horrible . . . I hope nothing happened or else it will be a big hunting job. (p. 546)

After another fifteen minutes in which the patient had changed the subject to problems he had experienced with his students, their abilities, and related issues, the analyst made the following interpretation: "Your earlier thoughts about the cleaning lady which occurred to you on the way here and your worry over losing her make me think that they may be connected with my upcoming absence for the next two weeks, starting next Monday" (p. 546).

Ramzy implies that his interpretation follows logically from the material (p. 548), but there are many other explanations for the patient's concern. These include first, the discovery, just before the analytic hour, that the cleaning lady had not arrived; and second, his previous experience with a cleaning lady's absence, which turned out to be a prelude to her moving away. From the standpoint of formal logic, we can find many reasons to dispute Ramzy's conclusion that the patient's extended worry about his cleaning lady is a derivative of his concern about the analyst's upcoming vacation. Nevertheless, his remark is not atypical of many clinical interventions. An interpretation is often under-determined by the evidence for the simple reason that timing is sometimes more important than logic, and if the analyst were to wait until he had assembled an airtight case, the remark would lose its relevance. The lion, as Freud once told us, only leaps once. What is more, an interpretation of this kind is often made for heuristic reasons in an effort to acquaint the patient with the possibility that manifest content may sometimes conceal significant latent content, and that awareness of both levels can enrich our understanding of any utterance.

But what is permissible in a clinical setting is not so easily tolerated in the public world of evidence and theory. It would appear that because the clinician has grown accustomed to drawing conclusions from small numbers of cases, he is less sensitized to the perils of this kind of thinking in a more scientific arena. He finds it too easy to assume that a handful of instances is sufficient to document a thesis. When we consider that the five cases described by Waugaman (Mr. A., Mrs. B., Mr. C., Mr. E., and Mr. G.) are a sample many times larger than what is normally assembled to make an interpretation, we begin to understand why he may have felt that his conclusion was supported by adequate evidence. But as we have indicated, five cases out of fifteen thousand (three thousand analysts times five cases) is only .03 percent of the total population—hardly a significant figure.

Another consequence of moving from a clinical to a scientific arena was briefly discussed in Chapter 3. In the clinical setting, the analyst is accustomed to basing his arguments on a coherence theory of truth, but once he decides to publish his findings, he feels he must appeal to the correspondence theory. As a result, he transforms a set of suggestive and original observations (such as the use of parents' first names by patients) into a general law ("Using the parent's first name unconsciously signifies an oedipal transgression"—Waugaman, 1990, p. 168). The law as stated seems to be unconditional and as intolerant of exception as, say, the law of gravity. The author/analyst seems to feel that by stating his findings in this fashion, he makes them more scientific and therefore more convincing. The contrary is probably more apt to be true. Unconditional laws of this kind only invite counterexamples, and a single negative instance is sufficient to demolish the strongest rule—the more general the law, the more easily it can be disconfirmed. At the least, this kind of unconditional wording invites skepticism and disbelief, and raises serious questions about the author's training in inductive logic.

The topic of Waugaman's paper is interesting in another connection: it points up the negative consequences of our anecdotal data base. We may not agree that the use of parents' first names necessarily represents an oedipal transgression, but Waugaman's clinical material makes it seem evident that this behavior may represent a significant transition point in the analytic process and that it can serve as an easily identified marker that lends itself particularly well to computer processing. But if we wanted to explore his hypothesis further, we would be frustrated by the anecdotal nature of the larger psychoanalytic data base. Suppose we picked one hundred case reports at random and looked for data on parents' first names. Our failure to find any mention of the issue would not necessarily indicate that it did not occur, only that it was not an issue that concerned the author. Because each clinical report is incomplete, it is almost useless as a basis for testing any hypothesis other than that originally formulated by the author. Our knowledge is limited by his horizon.

Evidence or Rhetoric?

A close inspection of Waugaman's paper gives us an opportunity to return to the role played by rhetoric in the typical psychoanalytic argument. The reader is told (in the abstract of the paper) that "patient's spontaneous disclosure of a parent's name is frequently associated with appearance of core conflicts . . . Using a parent's first name has the unconscious implication of incest, since one is doing something which one's other parent but not oneself is allowed to do" (1990, p. 167). Neither of these conclusions is supported by the evidence provided in the report. Their power to persuade the reader lies, therefore, not with logic but with rhetoric. To the extent that the reader is convinced by the argument, he is a victim of *argument by authority, hyperbole,* and *metaphor*—three well-known rhetorical devices. The conclusion is unrelated to the weight of the evidence.

The rhetorical voice, in this instance, masks the evidential voice because it makes us feel that we know the full meaning of using parents' first names when in fact we know only one possible interpretation of this behavior. Any satisfactory account of this phenomenon would need to collect dozens of instances from a large sample of additional patients and use these data to show that, in a significantly large number of cases, the use of parents' first names carried a particular perhaps even an oedipal—implication. The chances are good that several sets of meanings would be found, together with a large number of unexplained occurrences. But there is no precedent for this kind of evaluation in the psychoanalytic literature, and it is here that we see most clearly the way in which Freud's fascination with the specimen has contaminated subsequent research. It is hard to think of an example of current psychoanalytic research that is guided more by the clinical data than by the underlying theory.

In the face of the marginal evidence provided in the average clinical account, the rhetorical voice takes over. It is all too easy to use hyperbole, metaphor, metalepsis, and argument by authority to drown out the lack of evidence and persuade the doubtful reader that another derivative of the oedipal taboo—or some other favorite axiom—has been uncovered. This type of conclusion not only seems to add to our clinical wisdom, it implicitly strengthens the case for the essential truth of accepted psychoanalytic theory. But the case is more rhetorical than evidential, and it raises larger questions about the way in which a doubtful theory can be maintained through hopeful arguments and happy examples.

Not only is there no evidence in the Waugaman paper to support an oedipal interpretation, but the more fascinating implications of the phenomenon are being pushed aside in the rush to document a standard explanation. From the examples cited in the article, there seems no doubt that when and where a patient uses a parent's first name carries a great deal of clinical significance about the patient and must also contain important information about the transference. We can easily infer that the patient who never used his mother's first name, always referring to her as "the mother," was not exactly close to her, and may, as a consequence of this experience, have difficulty in other intimate relationships as well (see Waugaman, 1990, p. 171). We would like to know whether his use of first names changed with the course of treatment, both inside and outside the hour, but unfortunately this information is not provided. D. W. Winnicott also describes a patient who, three weeks before an interruption in the analysis, spoke of difficulty in using first names (p. 169). We may wonder if this material emerged because of the impending separation and could therefore be regarded as an indicator of the transference. What happened with respect to his pattern of naming behavior once the analysis was resumed? Once again, we are not told.

In this and other instances, questions raised by the clinical data are suppressed in favor of questions raised by the theory. The richness of observations collected by Waugaman provides us with a fascinating array of possibilities that could be properly explored only in a paper ten times longer than the one he has written. Instead, the bulk of the implied questions are left unanswered because of his *a priori* conviction that the use of parents' first names represents an oedipal transgression, because the sample size is usually too small to draw any kind of conclusion, and because Waugaman repeatedly commits what might be called the Clinician's Fallacy: he continues to believe that contiguity implies cause. We have seen that this error derives from one of the medieval similitudes. We now realize that it chokes off the collection of further data, because each new example becomes a covering law. No provision is made for the possibility that many co-occurrences may be entirely coincidental.

Embarrassing questions of this kind lie at the heart of any evidential investigation, yet they can be dismissed with no trouble once the author puts on his rhetorical hat. Then numbers are immaterial, sample size is unimportant, and the ringing tones of the argument matter more than the unsightly details of the raw data.

Can this paper be taken as a representative sample of clinical reporting? Regrettably, the answer is yes, and the implications are troubling. Largely because we have no adequate model of the way in which clinical evidence can be lawfully and systematically analyzed to frame and test hypotheses, author/analysts tend to fall back on Freud's anecdotal style and trust to a combination of happy example and persuasive utterance to convince the reader. But if the result rests more on rhetoric than on evidence, we must raise the question of whether the average case report is more campaign document than scientific investigation.

In a recent review of the case study method focusing in particular on the Rat Man and the Wolf Man, Grünbaum sees "both patient histories as counterproductive advertisements" (1988, p. 656). It would seem that "just the evidence based on these clinical case history procedures continues to leave the major pillars of psychoanalysis poorly supported" (p. 657). Grünbaum has elsewhere argued for the need to generate extra-clinical tests of the central assumptions of the theory (see Grünbaum, 1984). But if Freud's original cases stand on dubious arguments, and if subsequent clinical investigations are more rhetorical than evidential, where are the grounds for these central assumptions, which should be tested outside of the clinical setting? Is there any reason to take seriously a set of hypotheses originally inspired by fortuitous specimens and subsequently reinforced by a collection of happy instances?

If we take Williams's paper (see Chapter 6) and Waugaman's paper as metaphors for the current state of clinical reporting, we also begin to realize why psychoanalytic knowledge has not advanced much beyond Freud's original formulations. So long as official theory is given precedence and used to organize and formulate the clinical observations, it stands to reason that *only* evidence in support of the theory will be reported. If theory comes before data, there is no room for the unexplained finding because there is no framework, by definition, into which it can be fitted. Once again we see an unhappy reversal of roles. Where the clinician in the clinical setting is often quite willing to let the facts lead him to a conclusion, however unexpected, in his role as author/analyst, he takes a more conservative position and lets theory decide the way.

The result is a barren literature filled with theoretical clichés, anecdotal observations, and bad science masquerading as explanation. Homage to the status quo degrades the standard of reasoning and the quality of argument. We have abandoned such inductive principles as the importance of reasoning from a large sample and the need for cross-validation of any hypothesis, no matter how attractive, and have fallen back on the fascination with the single specimen that corrupted science before the Baconian revolution.

Alternatives to Theory-Centered Reports

The use of rhetoric as a substitute for inductive logic can be described as the underside of narrative truth. Williams's paper on the reconstruction of a possible infantile seduction makes it appear as if Freud's original formulation has been validated and we have gained another reason for upholding the received theory. It makes it appear as if we understand in greater detail exactly what happened to the patient when he was left alone with the servants and how this event colored his later life. Waugaman's paper on the use of parents' first names makes it appear as if we understand its general meaning—that is, as a marker of oedipal transgression—and that we now understand its clinical significance.

But these are rhetorical conclusions that are presented as if they were the fruits of normal science, with no discussion of the glaring methodological shortcomings of the analyses or the one-sided nature of the conclusions. The failure to acknowledge these defects sets a precedent for other authors and gradually desensitizes everyone— authors and readers alike—to the ways in which the typical case report is largely fraudulent and misleading. Reasonable accounts, largely in the service of accepted theory, are substituted for stammering and incomplete explanations of fragmentary data that can be explained in a variety of different ways. Preliminary observations—such as Waugaman's paper—are presented as if they were final reports that translate a small sample of clinical happenings into a general law—a law that, *mirabile dictu,* supports and extends the accepted theory.

When narrative is substituted for inductive reasoning and rhetoric for formal logic, the reader finds himself persuaded for reasons that are essentially accidental and contingent but not usually necessary. I spoke earlier (see Chapter 3) of the fact that the clinician in his practice must make maximal sense of the material close to hand, weighing various alternatives in a way that makes the greatest sense of the known facts and produces the most reasonable explanation. He argues in the service of narrative truth. But when the same tactic is applied to published findings, persuasion (and therefore rhetoric) takes precedence over lawfulness. In the clutch of the clinical moment, the analyst has no time to gather further evidence or debate one explanation vis-à-vis another, although it is precisely this longer perspective that we demand of scientific publications. To the extent that the current literature is largely made up of interpretations rushed into print, the clinical and scientific roles have been reversed.

When the author/analyst transforms a small sample of interesting (but essentially unexplained) happenings into a general law, he is not only allowing his clinical experience to influence his scientific standards, he is also carrying out a theory-centered method of investigation. In this approach, the investigator concentrates on finding evidence that will support the theory at hand, and as we have pointed out, it is always possible to achieve positive findings if the researcher is sufficiently persevering. In a discussion of the "corrupting effects of the hypothesis-testing method," McGuire makes the following observation:

> It can be taken for granted that some set of circumstances can be found to confirm *any* expressible relationship, provided that the researcher has sufficient stubbornness, stage management skills, resources, and stamina sooner or later to find or construct a situational context in which the predicted relationship reliably emerges. (1983, pp. 15–16; italics mine)

To guard against this danger, Greenwald et al. (1986) have argued for an approach that concentrates on the conditions under which the phenomenon of interest will appear. Rather than collect further examples and run the risk that positive findings are corrupted by mere perseverance, they encourage the researcher to study the pattern of significant behavior and to understand how a particular happening may emerge in the context of observation. In the case of calling parents by their first names, a pattern-finding approach might look at the sequence of hours just preceding the first appearance of the name and formulate hypotheses that would account for that particular sequence. These could be cross-validated on similar sequences drawn from other parts of the analysis or from other treatments.

This approach has an obvious bearing on the way we present our clinical findings. Rather than simply list the positive instances of the phenomenon, Waugaman could have provided a sequence of sessions surrounding the first occurrence. From these data, he and his readers could draw conclusions about the possible reasons why the patient felt free to mention the name for the first time. These reasons would suggest one or more hypotheses. In the author's first example, the case of Mr. A., we are told that he "had been in analysis for two months when he mentioned his mother's first name . . . It was another year and a half before Mr. A. next mentioned his mother's name" (1990, p. 172). We are told that his mother's name was the same as that of the patient who preceded him and whom he would often see in the waiting room. This patient

> had become a maternal transference figure, long before Mr. A. had consciously recognized that his mother and this patient shared the same first name. The first time Mr. A. mentioned Miss Jones [the patient], he said she had been the only person in my waiting room who had ever made eye contact with him. When she struck up conversation with him for the first time, he noticed her name tag [but, presumably, did not mention his mother]. He went on to speak of his pattern of reacting to momentary happiness by reminding himself of some humiliating experience from the past. This pattern reminded him of his mother: when he did something she was proud of, she would use it to point out how bad he was at other times. (p. 173)

This material suggests that Mr. A.'s reference to Miss Jones is linked in several ways with reference to his mother, and we would assume that the former would serve as a substitute for the latter long before he recognized that they shared the same first name. We next wonder what factors prevented this information from coming into awareness and what conditions enabled it to be recognized. If we were able to study the sequence of hours preceding the second reference, we might have a better understanding of the changing balance of conscious and unconscious factors that made this possible. We have gone beyond collecting instances to asking, Under what conditions does the phenomenon take place?

It should be noted that this way of asking questions about the evidence is not too different from the way in which the good clinician listens to his patient. He often draws attention to the emergence of a given pattern as background for a particular piece of behavior. He always wonders (silently if not aloud) how *this* pattern corresponds to *that* pattern, what set of circumstances made it possible for a given memory or image to appear for the first time, why a given interpretation now has an effect when before it went unheard. These and similar questions stem from a research-centered, as opposed to a theory-centered, approach to the data and enable us to understand the conditions that permit a clinical pattern to emerge.

By writing for publication in the same way he talks to his patients, the clinician is not only doing what comes naturally, he is also taking advantage of one of the recent advances in the theory of evidence. It is more and more a matter of common agreement among philosophers of science that the sheer accumulation of positive findings, an approach known as confirmation-biased research (see Greenwald et al., 1986), is not sufficient to prove a theory. Not only does premature fascination with the theory make every finding seem relevant (much as a boy with a hammer sees the world as full of nails), but with only one goal in mind the researcher is frequently unable to see other possibilities. In a weak and largely metaphoric sense, it is probably true that the use of parents' first names does represent an oedipal transgression, but this should be seen more as a rhetorical comment than as a full-fledged explanation. An adequate account will only emerge when we understand the range of situations in which the first-name phenomenon is likely to appear, the typical sequence of happenings that precede it, and what it represents to the patient in his relationship to his parents and to his analyst. This is why "the more valuable information obtainable through empirical confrontation emerges from the pattern of contexts in which the predicted relationship obtains as contrasted with those in which the contrary relationship or none at all obtains" (McGuire, 1983, p. 16).

When only a list of positive instances is available, we usually have little or no understanding of the conditions under which they emerged; in other words, we have no way of accounting for this particular pattern of results. Under these conditions, the pattern that does emerge is probably a mixture of accidental and necessary conditions, but because we have no way of separating the two strands, we are left with a clinical happening that is often poorly understood and frequently difficult to replicate (see Greenwald et al., 1986, p. 226). But when attention is focused on the pattern of results and the conditions under which they occur, we begin to learn something about the surrounding conditions that make the target happening possible and have a clearer awareness of the role it plays in the larger clinical picture.

A careful reading of Waugaman's paper reveals a great deal of unexplored clinical wisdom, which strongly suggests that the meaning of the target symptom has not been adequately explored. We can see that the need to link the phenomenon to standard theory too hastily has tended to get in the way of other hypotheses and interfere with an open-minded assessment of all the possibilities. A similar comment can be made about Williams's paper, for it too is dominated by an overfascination with received theory. In both cases, too much theory gets in the way of the facts.

But the problem is more easily diagnosed than solved because of the nature of the clinical report. As I have already noted, the reader is not given ready access to clinical happenings that lie outside the focus of the report. The full context of the target happening is not available, and a completely new study would seem to be required in order to provide what is needed (and missing). It should be noted that this issue really has nothing to do with protecting the confidentiality of the patient; it is rather a matter of treating the reader as an equal partner in the research enterprise and granting him full access to all relevant data.

In his paper "The Normative Structure of Science," Merton (1973) tells us that normal science is governed by a set of understood norms that include *universalism* and *communality*. The first requires that knowledge claims be bound by pre-established, impersonal criteria that are by definition necessary and not contingent; they must agree with previously established knowledge. The second requires that research be available to any interested scientist.

The special problems of psychoanalytic research do not lie, as some would argue, in the peculiar nature of its evidence. They lie instead in the failure to adhere to these two norms of normal science. The failure to follow these precepts can be laid directly at Freud's door: a variety of reasons led him to try to limit access to psychoanalytic wisdom. From Freud's obvious reluctance to document the psychoanalytic method and provide clear illustrations of the effect of specific interpretations, Sulloway draws the implicit message that Freud was seeking to convince his readers that psychoanalysis simply could not be learned from case histories (1991, p. 271). He believes that the uneven cases were designed to "convince potential converts to learn [Freud's] methods by another route. That other route, as it was developed and perfected by Freud's social technology, was the training analysis" (p. 271). In other words, by failing to provide a public data base and by restricting access to psychoanalytic findings to such non-universal institutions as the training analysis and individualized supervision of control cases, Freud was able to control the dissemination and application of his discoveries. But there is no present need to continue this practice, no reason why public data and open discussion cannot be combined with traditional training procedures. We no longer fear that full disclosure of a sequence of clinical happenings will enable the reader to become an instant analyst, although it will put him in a better position to understand the target phenomenon and the conditions under which it seems to appear.

8 Theories of the Mind: Fact or Fiction?

It is not news that distinctions between fact and fiction are disappearing a little bit every day and that before the century is out they may be gone for good. Libraries and best-seller lists still have separate sections for the two categories, but they may be among the last holdouts. At Princeton University, John McPhee has for many years offered a course on the literature of fact, and Hayden White, in *Tropics of Discourse,* speaks of the "fictions of factual representation." When Stephen Hawking, the Cambridge cosmologist, was asked if he was a regular reader of science fiction, he answered, "I read a fair amount of science fiction in my teens. Now I write it, only I like to think it is science fact."

Just as distinctions between fact and fiction are rapidly becoming more arbitrary, similar worries surround the difference between theory and make-believe. Facts, it would seem, are rarely transparent, theory is never entirely data-driven, and observations are almost always theory-laden. Of course, theories claim to be about something real, but aside from that important proviso there is often little to distinguish them from fiction. On some occasions, to further complicate the picture, the terms of fiction make more precise reference to the real world than do the terms of science, just the opposite of our traditional belief. Whereas we used to think that "theoretical terms within a science can refer to real world events with sufficient precision that the propositions in which such terms are featured can be subjected to empirical assessment" (Gergen and Gergen, 1986, p. 23), we now realize that unambiguous reference is not so easy to establish.

When are the facts most often out of reach? What the Gergens (1986) have called the problem of the "vanishing object" becomes

164

especially critical when we focus on theories of the mind. Whereas early explanations of behavior invoked the heart, the pineal gland, and other more or less accessible body parts as the seat of the soul and the source of emotions and thought, we have tended, over the years, to leave the body behind and search for explanations in the stuff of the mind. And this stuff is, as we have seen in Chapter 4, notoriously hard to specify or examine—hence the appeal of metaphor. Our present emphasis on the (unavailable) stuff of the mind may, in fact, be the direct consequence of unsuccessful past dissections. During the eighteenth century, Dr. Benjamin Rush actually performed autopsies on patients who had died of grief and discovered, so he claimed, "congestion of, and inflammation of, the heart, with a rupture of its auricles and ventricles" (1812, p. 318). Diagnosis of a "broken heart," it would seem, was thereby directly confirmed! But as subsequent investigations began to cast doubt on this observation, we have been forced to look elsewhere for the causes of behavior. As our knowledge of anatomy has become more precise, we have tended to cast doubt on the role of the heart, the liver, and the spleen in generating feelings.

We begin to see how, precisely because of their concrete language, early theories of behavior could be directly disconfirmed by dissection and autopsy. But once we move our search to the region of the mind, we find that access to the facts becomes much more difficult; as a result, disconfirmation is largely out of reach and metaphors flourish in abundance. What Schafer has called the "mover of the mental apparatus" (1976, Chap. 5) no longer exists in any particular place, and theories take refuge in such things as the "forces of the mind," which cannot be measured. Thus we find Freud writing that "we seek not merely to describe and clarify phenomena, but to understand them as signs of an interplay of forces of the mind, as a manifestation of purposeful intentions working concurrently or in mutual opposition" (1916, p. 67).

More recent explanations have tended to take refuge in the unconscious, but as we have seen in Chapter 4, this is more a metaphor than a consensually validated referent. For Stanley Fish, the

unconscious is not a concept but a rhetorical device, a place holder which can be given whatever shape the polemical moment requires. If someone were to object to his interpretation of a particular detail, he could point for confirmation to the nature of the unconscious, and, if someone were to dispute the nature of the unconscious, he could point to the evidence of his interpretations; and all the while he could speak of himself as being "obliged" by constraints that were at once independent *of* him and assured independence *from* him of his patient and his reader. The rhetorical situation could not be more favorable. (1986, p. 936)

What has happened to language? Where Benjamin Rush could dissect the cadavers of patients who had died of grief and look for signs of congestion and inflammation in the cardiac auricles, the new theory of the unconscious was literally unfalsifiable. Because we are denied access to what is being described, we have no way to correct the original description. It may be sensed, as I noted in Chapter 4, as wildly extravagant or clearly impossible, but whatever reaction it inspires, it remains in force because it cannot be disproved. What was originally conceived as a model of the mind has become (in the minds of many) the standard explanation of how the mind works. This kind of metaphorical takeover draws its power both from the evocative quality of the images presented and from the fact that we have no direct access to the stuff of the mind. If we did, the "seething cauldron" would become as old-fashioned as the "broken heart."

Theories of the mind would seem to be particularly susceptible to fictional influence and metaphorical take-over because the stuff of the mind is largely out of reach. As a result, there are no reality constraints on our use of language. Because their data are largely invisible, theories of the mind are particularly susceptible to three major sources of influence: the prevailing scientific and literary Zeitgeist, the personal history of the theorist, and what might be called the contemporary root metaphor. Let us consider first the Zeitgeist.

Cultural Influences

For a particularly clear example of the way in which cultural context can influence theory, it is informative to examine theories of the two hemispheres of the brain and relate them to the countries in which they originated.

In Germany, united for the first time under the Prussian bureaucracy, most scientists described the brain as a set of functionally distinct departments; English medical writers, confronted with the psychiatric consequences of a class-based society, worried how the rational cortex could control lower, more primitive elements of the central nervous system. It was only in France, especially in the uncertain early years of the Third Republic, that anti-Catholic liberal scientists were determined to show that civilization and rationality resided necessarily on the Left, while decadence and mysticism were on the Right. (Pauley, 1988, p. 422)

For a more detailed example of the same kind of influence, we might consider the way in which the new science of archeology, in the last part of the nineteenth century, came to have such a significant influence on the form and content of Freud's theory of the mind. Malcolm Bowie describes the scene:

Archeology was for Freud the supreme combination of art and science and exerted a special fascination upon him throughout his career. And that career, we need hardly remind ourselves, spanned a golden age of archeological discovery: Schliemann was unearthing his many-layered Troy at Hissarlik during Freud's school and university years; Evans was exploring and then excavating Knossos during the period of Freud's self analysis and of his collaborative friendship with Breuer and Fliess; Freud was writing *The Ego and the Id* in the year Carnarvon and Carter discovered the tomb of Tutankhamen, and *The Future of an Illusion* and *Civilization and Its Discontents* during Woolley's excavation of Sumerian Ur. Freud was an avid reader of archeological memoirs and a spendthrift collector of antiquities. In a letter of 1931 to Stefan Zweig, he strove to correct Zweig's recently published portrait of him in the following terms: "Despite my much vaunted frugality I have sacrificed a great deal for my collection of Greek, Roman and Egyptian antiquities, have actually read more archeology than psychology, and . . . before the war and once after its end I felt compelled to spend every year at least several days or weeks in Rome." (1988, p. 18)

Archeology was widely discussed all during this period, but it was much more than a metaphor. It became a guiding model that strongly influenced Freud's belief in the persistent power of memory and his conception of the timeless unconscious. We are all familiar with the parallels he found between doing psychoanalysis and uncovering ruins. Not only did he try to take current fragments of memory and use them to reconstruct earlier happenings in the life of the patient, but he also saw a parallel between the age of a fragment and its state of preservation. One of the earliest expressions of this metaphor appears in his "Fragments of an Analysis of a Case of Hysteria":

In the face of the incompleteness of my analytic results, I had no choice but to follow the example of those discoverers whose good fortune it is to bring to the light of day after their long burial the priceless though mutilated relics of antiquity. I have restored what is missing, taking the best models known to me from other analyses; but, like a conscientious archeologist, I have not omitted to mention in each case where the authentic parts end and my constructions begin. (1905, p. 12)

And in similar vein, toward the end of his life, he wrote:

But just as the archeologist builds up the walls of the buildings from the foundations that have remained standing, determines the number and position of the columns from depressions in the floor and reconstructs the mural decorations and paintings from the remains found in the debris, so does the analyst proceed when he draws his inferences from the fragments of memories, from the associations and from the behavior of the subject of the analysis. (1937, p. 259)

Part of the appeal of the archeologist's discoveries lay in their remarkable preservation. Under certain conditions (as in the tomb of Tutankhamen), time seemed to have stopped; everything was just as it had been thousands of years before Christ. The parallels with the timeless unconscious seem obvious, and Freud treated the analogy as fact in the absence of any real evidence. "In mental life," he wrote, "nothing which has once been formed can perish . . . everything is somehow preserved and . . . in suitable circumstances it can once more be brought to light" (quoted in Bowie, p. 22).

Not only was everything preserved, but the facts were transparent and needed no interpretation. When the tomb of King Tut was uncovered, its significance was clearly obvious. It was headline news and its meaning was transparent. "Saxa loquuntur," Freud was fond of saying: Stones speak. We can argue that the archeological metaphor led directly to Freud's impatience with the need for evidence and his belief that observation was everything. Out of this impatience grew our present case study tradition, which relies largely on anecdote and argument by authority. If facts are transparent, there is no need for interpretation, no need for peer review of the evidence, no need for any kind of archival collection or data base.

Psychoanalysis was not only similar to archeology—it went one better: "Whereas the archeologist's material may be complete, or broken beyond repair, the psychoanalyst's is indestructible. This theme, which has cautious beginnings (the lesson of Freud's antiquities as taught to the Rat Man was merely that 'what was unconscious was relatively unchangeable'), was to develop into a guiding principle of clinical observation" (Bowie, 1988, p. 22). The analyst uses the same model but "works under more favorable conditions than the archeologist," because the latter may be faced with the destruction of significant objects, whereas for the analyst, "all of the essentials are preserved; even things that seem completely forgotten are present somehow and somewhere, and have merely been buried and made inaccessible to the subject" (Freud, 1937, p. 260).

If facts are transparent and meaning is obvious, there is no room for individual interpretation or influence. Because of its appeal to hard fact, the archeological model protected Freud from any charge of suggestion. If he could claim that his method allowed him to make contact with the actual past, then he could defend himself against the charge of supplying some of the answers. It is worth noting that Freud's most ambitious attempts at reconstruction, described in the Wolf Man case, took place at a time when he was defending his theory against competing formulations. "The primary significance of the [Wolf Man case] at the time of its publication," writes Strachey in his introduction, "was clearly the support it provided for his criticisms of Adler and more especially of Jung. Here was conclusive evidence to refute any denial of infantile sexuality" (Freud, 1918, p. 5; editor's note).

The archeological metaphor was not only a useful model of the mind; it also carried enormous rhetorical clout because it brought with it an appeal to certainty that was hard to resist. If all memories are skulls and mummies, we are back to psychic bedrock at long last. The metaphor is so persuasive, we lose sight of the fact that it is largely fictitious. And what is more, as Bowie has pointed out, the archeological model carries the strong suggestion that psychoanalysis is theory-free and that observation is king. This suggestion is largely fiction, but fiction so well disguised that we fail to realize we are in the hands of a master storyteller.

So much for the influence of one part of the Zeitgeist on Freud's theory of the mind. It seems more than likely that psychoanalysis would look quite different if Freud had lived only fifty years earlier, before any of the great excavations had taken place. And this influence was in no manner uncharacteristic; in any number of instances, the language of explanation has been borrowed from the culture of its time. Early theories, as we have seen, drew on the developing knowledge of anatomy and the belief that emotions were based in the heart and other body organs. By the late nineteenth century, the stuff of the mind was being conceived by Freud in terms of the mechanical, energy-conserving metaphors of the industrial revolution. In the late twentieth century, we have moved on to the computer and artificial intelligence for the source of our language (for example, parallel and serial processing and Gardner's theory of mental modules; see Gardner, 1983). The influence of contemporary culture is not surprising, but it remains somewhat troublesome, because this tendency suggests that the source of any particular theory of the mind is more fortuitous than otherwise and that the choice of metaphor does not necessarily indicate any specific insight into the workings of the mind.

Edward Sampson (1981) has pointed to the way in which current models of the mind draw their inspiration from the technological aspects of our culture, which stress technical mastery and active control over nature. "We err," he writes, "by routinely assuming the forms of empirical-analytic science (the technical interest) as our implicit framework for understanding human life and behavior" (p. 741). These preferences become even more suspicious when we see them as largely arbitrary. If we have no direct knowledge of the stuff of the mind, then we must find terms from some other domain, and the choice of domain may tell us more about our value system than about the object being described.

Personal Influences

If theories of the mind are as much fiction as fact, it is not surprising that one important source of make-believe would be the personal history of the scientist. The psychobiography of leading theorists of the mind is a field only just now coming into its own, and to date, it promises more than it has delivered. Even if the promise is significant, it remains hard to validate. While it stands to reason that the personal history of the theorist should influence the structure of his creation, it has not been easy to establish clear links between biographical details and the form and content of finished theory.

The hypothesis is best stated by Stolorow and Atwood: "It is our contention that the subjective world of the theorist is inevitably translated into his metapsychological conceptions and hypotheses concerning human nature, limiting the generality of his theoretical constructions and lending them a coloration expressive of his personal existence as an individual" (1979, p. 17). A reasonable expectation, one would think, but the links between the life and work of such theorists as Freud, Jung, Rank, and Wilhelm Reich are not that convincing. The pattern matches discovered by Stolorow and Atwood are plausible but not particularly compelling, and the link between biography and theory is certainly not inevitable.

Nevertheless, some details are quite striking. "Many of Freud's most unsettling ideas," writes Gay (1988), "drew on acknowledged, or covert, autobiographical sources. He exploited himself freely as a witness and made himself into the most informative of his patients" (p. 90). We know that Freud was the son of a young mother of twenty-one and a father twenty years older, that he was the firstborn son of this marriage, and that the next-oldest child, Julius, was born eleven months later and died when Freud was nineteen months old. Something of the special feelings that go with being the firstborn can be sensed in the following confession on a return visit to his birthplace in 1931: "Deep within me, covered over, there still lives that happy child from Freiberg, the first-born son of a youthful mother, who had received the first indelible impressions from this air, from this soil" (quoted in Gay, 1988, p. 9).

The family constellation of older father, younger mother, and (for a time) only child, as we have already made clear, seems made to order for an oedipal interpretation. We know the importance of the oedipal triangle in Freud's clinical theory, and it is tempting to argue that, had he been born into a different family constellation, this hypothesis might not have been given the emphasis it has received. Quite a different theory might have resulted if his parents had been separated early in life (which was the case with Jung, for example, whose mother was hospitalized soon after he was born).

The circumstances of Freud's early life must have sensitized him to the possibilities for oedipal rivalry. The question to be considered is whether he gave them a significance that goes beyond the norm. When we shift from the discovery of the Oedipus complex to its application, the influence of personal events becomes harder to follow. "What must matter to the student of psychoanalysis," writes Gay, "is ultimately not whether Freud had (or imagined) an Oedipus complex, but whether his claim that it is the complex through which *everyone must pass* can be substantiated by independent observers or ingenious experiments" (p. 90, italics mine). And while it may be true, as Gay argues, that "Freud did not regard his own experiences as automatically valid for all humanity" (p. 90), their evidential standing rather quickly changed from hypotheses to axioms (see Spence, 1987). As Gay admits in a later passage, "the private provenance of his convictions would not inhibit Freud from developing a theory . . . about the ubiquitous family drama with its ever-varied yet largely predictable plot of wishes, gratifications, frustrations, and losses, many of them unconscious" (p. 90). Far from preventing such a theory, I would argue that his private convictions may well have fueled it.

A specific private event may sensitize a theorist to certain aspects of experience and place him in a better position to make sense out of certain life events. It may also bring with it a certain feeling of inevitability that is translated into theoretical rigidity. Since it happened to me, goes the unacknowledged argument, it must happen to Everyman; since it happened to me, no one dares challenge it. We begin to see the grounds for a troubling link between biographical detail and theoretical dogma. The parts of the theory that the author feels most reluctant to change—even in the face of disconfirming facts—may well be those that spring directly from some childhood source. We might wonder whether it was Freud's personal investment in his theory that made him so reluctant to accept any kind of correction.

A related question can also be asked: does biographical overdetermination play a part in narrative persuasion? In other words, could it be that the parts of the theory that carry the most influence—from either a rhetorical or a scientific point of view—are those that stem directly from the thinker's childhood? Consider the far-reaching appeal of the oedipal complex. Does it rest entirely on the Greek myth, or is it given some special urgency by Freud's personal experience, which finds its optimal expression in particular parts of his theory? Raising questions of this kind brings us closer to the way in which early experience may not only compel a particular view of the world but give wings to its expression and cause others to be persuaded of its truth.

Whatever the role of the personal past on the evolving theory of the mind, it seems clear that all theorists commit some form of the personal fallacy: what seems true for the thinker must (they think) be true of all people. We have noted how theories of the mind, because they

are cut off from the stuff they are describing, are particularly susceptible to extraneous influence. We now realize that there is another side
to the problem. The conviction that stems from personal experience
may so impress the theorist that he sees no reason to check his facts
against the data systematically. And even though Gay argues in support of his open stance and claims that Freud "tested his notions
against the experiences of his patients . . . against the psychoanalytic
literature . . . [and] spent years working over, refining, revising, his
generalizations" (1988, p. 90), the oedipal complex rather quickly
assumed the status of a universal finding in a form not too different
from its earliest formulation. The combination of ambiguous evidence
and a committed theorist who is working out of significant and not
completely remembered life experience makes for a theory that does
not lend itself easily to revision. If favorite rhetorical devices have been
added to the mix, it becomes all the more difficult to revise and
rewrite.

Underlying Root Metaphors

We have seen that, because their referents are largely unseen, theories
of the mind are particularly susceptible to narrative mischief. This
problem becomes particularly acute when we turn to theories of infant
development for the obvious reason that we are dealing, in the early
stages of life, with a mind that has no language and therefore cannot
tell us whether our theories are right or wrong. We will consider one
well-known theory of this kind and go on to examine the underlying
root metaphors that seem to support its narrative structure.

The theory in question is the one associated with Margaret Mahler,
which describes what has been called the psychological birth of the
human infant. This birth begins with an autistic phase from about one
to six months during which "the infant spends most of his day in a
half-sleeping, half-waking state: he wakes principally when hunger or
other need tensions . . . cause him to cry, and sings or falls asleep again
when he is satisfied" (Mahler, Pine, and Bergman, 1975, p. 41). He
next moves into a symbiotic phase in which he "begins dimly to per-
ceive need satisfaction as coming from some need-satisfying part-
object—albeit still from within the orbit of the omnipotent symbiotic
dual unity" of mother and child (p. 46). "The essential feature of sym-
biosis is hallucinatory or delusional . . . omnipotent fusion with the

representation of the mother and, in particular, the delusion of a common boundary between two physically separate individuals" (p. 45).

Next comes what is called the period of differentiation, which is divided into three subphases: hatching, practicing, and rapproachment. In the first, or hatching, phase, "we came to recognize . . . a certain new look of alertness, persistence and goal-directness. We have taken this look to be a behavioral manifestation of 'hatching' . . . [although] it is difficult to define with specific criteria" (p. 54). In the rapproachment subphase, the observers were struck by two forms of behavior—shadowing and darting away. These activities "indicate both his wish for reunion with the love object and his fear of re-engulfment by it. One can continually observe in the toddler a 'warding off' pattern directed against impingement upon his recently achieved autonomy . . . At the very height of his mastery, toward the end of the practicing period, it had already begun to dawn on the junior toddler that the world is *not* his oyster, that he must cope with it more or less 'on his own' " (p. 78).

During this phase, the mother changes in a significant way: "At around 15 months, we noticed an important change in the quality of the child's relationship to his mother. During the practicing period . . . mother was 'home base' to which the child returned often in times of need—need for food, need for comforting, or need for 'refueling' when tired or bored . . . Somewhere around 15 months, mother was no longer just 'home base.' She seemed to be turning into a person with whom the toddler wished to share his ever-widening discoveries of the world" (p. 90).

We have just summarized a widely cited theory of early development. What gives it its special appeal? Part of its persuasive power arises from such specific metaphors as *hatching, shadowing, rapproachment, home base,* and *refueling;* although these figures of speech clearly go beyond the data, they do so in engaging ways. But it seems unlikely that language alone would be enough to account for Mahler's popularity. Her theory draws its particular strength from two underlying root metaphors: the myth of the young hero and the myth of the New World discoverer.

The myth of the hero has a long tradition in American fiction. It is one of our most cherished stories and encompasses our most popular heroes. Beginning with Huck Finn, we move on to Henry Fleming *(The*

Red Badge of Courage), to Billy Budd, and to Eugene Gant *(Look Homeward, Angel),* and end up with Holden Caulfield *(Catcher in the Rye).* Leaving home at a young age to learn the lessons of the world, each of these heroes finds his own method of making each trip a little longer and returning to home base less and less often. Mahler's formulation provides an interesting counterpoint to this analysis of the *Red Badge of Courage:*

> Crane's main theme is the discovery of self, that unconscious self, which, when identified with the inexhaustible energies of the group, enables man to understand the deep forces that have shaped man's destiny. The progressive movement of the hero, as in all myth, is that of *separation, initiation, and return* . . . he is transformed through a series of rites and revelations into a hero. (Hart, 1962, p. 264; italics mine)

Mahler's toddler leaves his mother in progressively longer voyages of discovery, voyages that are clearly necessary for defining his character through repeated separations, which result in what might be called the birth of the hero. This particular version of the psychological birth of the infant is rooted in a very American story, which resonates with any number of past presences, both real and make-believe. This story or myth places special emphasis on individuality, separation, and the importance of learning from experience. We hear overtones of John Dewey and the frontier spirit. It seems to capture, in microcosm, the coming of age of an American male. According to Leslie Fiedler,

> The Good Bad Boy is, of course, America's vision of itself, crude and unruly in his beginnings, but endowed by his creator with an instinctive sense of what is right. Sexually as pure as any milky maiden, he is a roughneck all the same, at once potent and submissive, made to be reformed by the right woman . . . In our national imagination, two freckle-faced boys, arm in arm, fishing poles over their shoulders, walk toward the river . . . They are on the lam, we know, from Aunt Polly and Aunt Sally and the widow Douglas and Miss Watson, from golden-haired Becky Thatcher, too—from all the reduplicated female symbols of "sivilization" . . .
>
> Not only does [Twain] disavow physical passion, refusing the Don Juan role traditional for European writers; but he downgrades even the Faustian role incumbent on American authors. In him, the diabolic outcast becomes the "little devil," not only comical but cute, a child who will outgrow his mischief, or an imperfect adult male, who

needs the "dusting off" of marriage to a good woman . . .

The myth which Twain creates is a myth of childhood, rural, sex-less, yet blessed in its natural Eden by the promise of innocent love, and troubled by the shadow of bloody death. (1966, pp. 271–273)

Coming back to Mahler's theory, we begin to understand some of its appeal and its ability to create in us the sense that this is how things really are. Every child, we are told, behaves like a young Henry Fleming or Huck Finn. Every infant is born with a natural desire to leave his mother and make his mark on the dining room, the living room, the kitchen, or the bedroom. His wanderlust carries him into what Mahler has called his "ever-widening discoveries of the world." Venture far enough and you return a hero, loved by your mother and proud of yourself. Individuality is not only sanctioned, it is the American way, the road to becoming a man and conquering the world.

This quotation brings us to a related root metaphor: Columbus and the discovery of America. The clue is provided by Louise Kaplan in her layman's version of Mahler's theory:

On his third voyage to the New World, Columbus suddenly with-drew. He fled back to Hispaniola. He returned to home base. It is said that as he confronted the downward-flowing turbulence of the Orinoco he was overcome with the sense that he must be mounting toward the Garden of Eden . . . He reckoned that he must have arrived at the foot of the Holy Mountain, the paradise with its for-bidden secrets . . .

And like Columbus, we also pause at the borders of our new worlds. We hesitate. We return to base. We draw up new maps. We try to reconcile the old geometry with the new calculus that is still only a vision. We chart our journeys with fluttering heartbeats and quivering apprehensions. (1978, pp. 246–247)

Discovery can become tinged with both excitement and fear; the nursery becomes the headwaters of the Orinoco. The early years of childhood are not merely the training ground for a hero—they are heroic in themselves. The feat of the child when he strays too far becomes the equivalent of the terror Columbus felt when he found himself getting too close to Eden. When he sets out again on a longer journey, we cheer because he has looked this terror in the face and stared it down.

Given much less emphasis in Mahler's theory—all but ignored—is the Becky Thatcher view of the world with its virtues of staying put, of clinging, of remaining by the mother's side. Even though these are also frequent behaviors of the young girl child, they are little discussed. When we realize that these virtues, more often associated with a feminine coming of age, are minimized in Mahler's theory, we begin to see more clearly the importance of the myth of the male hero and the significance of this particular root metaphor.

Mahler's theory also does something else: it peoples the world with little men thinking adult thoughts. Mahler speaks of omnipotence, persistence, and goal-directedness, but these are hardly infantile traits. Does a child "wish for reunion with his love-object"? Does he relish his newfound autonomy? This sounds like the analyst speaking. Mahler's theory takes the baby talk out of childhood and tempts us into thinking that even though the toddler cannot speak, he is thinking grown-up thoughts and engaged in grown-up actions. Another reason for Mahler's appeal may be that she pushes the toddler into adulthood.

How Theory Obstructs Progress

As we begin to find ways in which the current Zeitgeist, the specific background of the theorist, and felicitious root metaphors shape the form and content of a particular theory, we begin to sense another kind of danger. Not only is the theory arbitrarily dominated by a certain view of the world, but by its very existence it stands in the way of new theories and new observations. So long as we are inspired by the myth of the hero, for example, we find it all but impossible to take note of what is really going on in the playroom. Instead of providing epistemic access to the clinical happenings of the nursery in all of their seemingly irrational complexity, the myth-ridden theory tends to blind us to the unexpected and to smooth over the facts that do not fit our scenarios, and tempts us to invent other facts that do. A persuasive theory, in short, can make us "see" what is not there at all.

An arbitrary (and therefore partly fictitious) theory also obstructs because it traps us into testing irrelevancies. I have noted the appeal by Greenwald and his collaborators (1986) to stop the mindless accumulation of happy examples. Any theory, they point out, can be patched up to fit the facts; any body of data sufficiently large can be sifted over to find supporting instantiations. They suggest that more time be spent on approving and disapproving of theories than on proving or disproving them. Approval and disapproval take us into the questions of fact and fiction that are central to this discussion. What has been primarily a literary, deconstructive analysis of Mahler's theory has highlighted some disturbing parallels with the myth of the young hero in American fiction. A critical review of Freud's archeological metaphor has uncovered some troubling links to the scientific Zeitgeist of the nineteenth century. A review of the Oedipus theory in the light of Freud's upbringing raises disturbing questions about the extent to which it is more a theory about Freud than about man in general.

Discovery of these connections makes it clear, first of all, that theories are never culture-free, and it may be their links to crucial parts of the Zeitgeist that make them last long after their prime, not their ability to explain the facts. We have seen that it is always possible to find evidence to support a given proposition. But confirming data will never tell us that our theory is phallocentric and sentimentally tied to a rich lode of American folklore, and that for this reason alone it needs to be viewed with suspicion.

We have viewed theories of the mind conventionally as if they were provisional descriptions of what is happening inside the head, hypothetical and metaphorical at the start, but subject to greater refinement as the facts become clear. Now we realize that they may always remain largely metaphorical and therefore not subject to disconfirmation. But the very fact that theories of the mind are also cultural products gives us another way of assessing their worth. As we become aware of their narrative and rhetorical loading and the way in which their resonance with the Zeitgeist gives them easy access to our approval, we can also better defend against them. If we think of theories of the mind as representative fictions that should be discussed partly in narrative and rhetorical terms, we may be better positioned to separate their emotional appeal from their scientific usefulness. This stance allows us to distance ourselves from the theory, to look critically at its language as separate from its content, and to become more aware of the factors underlying its staying power.

A concentrated hermeneutic reading would help us better understand a theory's ability to survive in the scientific marketplace. Some theories of the mind have a fascination and staying power that seems to be out of all proportion to their relation to the data or to their capacity to explain. As is well known, not all theories come to grief when the evidence goes against them. It has been the fashion to assume that if a theory is still with us, it must somehow be in touch with the facts; it must be telling part of the truth. Now we would suspect that this last clause applies primarily to *narrative* truth. Staying power, it would seem, has more to do with narrative smoothing, rhetorical appeal, and the extent to which its central concepts and root metaphors reduplicate critical features of the Zeitgeist.

The Need for Consensual Validation

But hermeneutic and deconstructive readings can only go so far. While they may sensitize us to the ways in which a fashionable theory too suspiciously resembles its author's background or the culture's root metaphors, such readings will not correct flawed concepts or give us better ways of talking about clinical happenings. Sooner or later, the central concepts must be exposed to the test of the marketplace, subjected to the traditional cross-validation and replication expected of any empirical science.

These cross-checks would seem particularly necessary when we are dealing with theories of the mind. Because the critical referents are largely out of reach, and because the shape of the theory can be so easily influenced by idiosyncratic factors in the personal background and surrounding culture of its author, it seems all the more necessary to confront theory with as much data as can be conveniently gathered. Whether or not the theory is truly general can never be determined by armchair inspection, because all but the worst ideas have a plausible face validity; only by looking at large numbers of cases from a variety of different sources can we determine whether a theory has scientific standing over and above its rhetorical appeal.

But this move—from an Aristotelian fascination with the single specimen to a Galilean concern with multiple occurrences—has been slow in coming for reasons I have noted in the preceding chapters. Even one hundred years after Freud's initial discoveries, it is by no means certain that the majority of analysts see the need for this kind of transition. I noted in Chapter 4 that despite the fact that such a move seems necessary and just, it must fight against the suggestive and persuasive rhetorical voice of psychoanalysis, which keeps telling us, in a variety of ways that standard theory is explanation enough, that new arguments would only detract from its majesty, and that challenges to the theory raise more questions about the changes than about what is being changed. As we become aware of the ways in which the standard theory is linked to significant themes in the culture and to important features of the author's personality, we see another reason why change is slow and meets with so much resistance. To say that perhaps Freud's theory is more true of him than of the whole human race would seem like another way of diminishing his stature and marginalizing his contribution. It would also be saying, in effect, that the heroic effort that made up the self-analysis was significantly flawed and can no longer be celebrated as an intellectual achievement of mythic proportions.

So long as standard theory is intermixed with the familiar story of its creator and his personal strengths and weaknesses on the one hand, and rooted in significant pieces of the culture on the other, it can never be treated dispassionately as a set of concepts, axioms, and hypotheses in continual need of validation and reformulation. The rhetorical voice is embedded not only in familiar metaphor but in Freud's favorite analogies; even though we are beginning to recognize some of his more flagrant rhetorical moves (with the help, for example, of Fish, 1986, and Mahony, 1987), we are far from casting off his persuasive appeal. Even his most articulate critic, Adolf Grünbaum, at the end of his closely reasoned attack on the philosophical foundations of the theory, finds himself calling for the extra-clinical validation of Freud's most important hypotheses: "Despite the poverty of the clinical credentials," he tells us, "it may perhaps still turn out that Freud's brilliant imagination was actually quite serendipitous for psychopathology or the understanding of some subclass of slips" (1984, p. 278). To come down on the side of Freud after spending nearly three hundred pages finding flaws in his clinical and logical arguments is clearly a sign of the power of the rhetorical voice. We look in vain to find reasons for this change of tone. Finding none, we must conclude that Grünbaum, like the rest of us, is susceptible to the appeal of rhetoric and to Freud's masterful powers of persuasion.

It may well turn out that standard theory will never be replaced— or will at least remain the same for some time to come. But the reasons are rhetorical and sentimental, not evidential. So long as we continue (as in Gay's biography and the recent centennial testimonials) to celebrate the heroic story of Freud's life and work and to recognize the many ways in which the two are entangled, it will never be possible to separate his ideas from his view of the world and from his passion for psychoanalysis. His life is still, as in Gay's subtitle, "a life for our time," and the force of his presence and the specific effect of his language compels us—again, for rhetorical reasons—not only to respect his theory but to treat it as sacred. Even as the evidence mounts that it is unsupported by the clinical findings, that it is the product of a specific man, working in a specific cultural period, and of a specific developmental history, and that the evidence for its therapeutic value is still problematic—even in the face of all these questions, we still respond to its appeal.

In view of such powerful, irrational factors, it seems likely that no amount of contrary evidence will bring about a significant change in standard theory. I noted (in Chapter 4) our preference for the now-familiar phrasing of the *Standard Edition*. New findings will necessarily spoil some of the sweeping sentences that are now part of our psychoanalytic and cultural heritage. Exceptions to this or that general formulation—to many of the sweeping statements quoted in my Introduction—will necessarily make the theory more hedged about with restrictive clauses and, as a result, less literary and (very likely) less readable. We begin to realize that theory speaks with both a factual and a rhetorical voice, and we may not be able to improve the first if it means giving up the second.

The fact that, at the moment, evidence is not decisive speaks once again to the power of the rhetorical voice. A focus on this power suggests a possible sequence of events for the future. When the copyright runs out, there will almost certainly be a new translation of Freud, and this new version will almost certainly combine familiar phrases with new formulations, familiar concepts with new approximations. As the present Strachey translation fades into the past, we will be released from its familiar and persuasive voice and in a position to look more realistically at the clinical facts. Freed from this long-standing influence, we will be more ready, it would seem, to let the evidence speak with its own voice and more willing to accept change when it seems demanded by the facts. But until this day comes, the standard theory, because of its familiarity and its rhetorical advantage, will take precedence over any new set of clinical happenings, no matter how reliable or consensually validated.

When a new translation comes into being and the language changes, we will hear Freud through the new voice of science, and this implicit air of objectivity will give us permission, as it were, to take a more searching view of the evidence. When this time comes the status of the clinical happening will seem to change overnight, and the relation between data and theory will come to agree more with what we find in the other sciences. A new translation is also likely to benefit from more open discussion of the standing of the standard theory and to correct many of the wrongs in the current professional literature. But it is important to note that rhetorical change must come first. Only when our rhetoric changes will what Francis Bacon called the "idols of the marketplace" give way to more enduring formulations.

9   A New Evidential Surface

As an example of the way in which imprecise language has contributed to theoretical stalemate, it may be useful to consider a recent discussion of the topic of the analytic surface (Seelig, 1993). A panel of analysts paid much attention to the concept of surface and its various meanings, but even though the discussion made it clear that *surface* is not an "official" term in psychoanalysis (it does not appear in any of the specialized glossaries; see Seelig, 1993, p. 179), and even though precise meaning remains elusive, the panel nevertheless (and somewhat surprisingly) concluded that it was a useful concept that could be helpful in teaching technique (p. 186) and that it was critically connected to the central aims of treatment. One of the panelists stated that "the goal of analysis is to extend the patient's self-knowledge as much beyond the surface as possible" (p. 180). But how can this be done if the concept remains undefined? When the chair concluded the panel by thanking everyone for a "stimulating and rewarding experience," was he merely being polite, or did he feel that something had in fact been learned? The second option seems hard to credit.

Let us consider some of the definitions of surface that panel members presented. For Warren Poland, surface "is the place to begin but not the place to end"; put another way, it "lies in the affective engagement of the two partners in the uniquely structured analytic setting" (p. 181). He distinguished *topographic* from *metaphoric* and *dynamic* surface. For Miriam Goldberger, the surface can be located at the place where the defenses are active (p. 182). Henry Smith discussed the "phenomenal surface" (p. 184) and distinguished the patient's perception of the surface from the analyst's. Dale Boesky, the panel discussant, called attention to a "neglected surface," defined as "all that the patient could tell us if asked, but has not yet told us" (p. 185). Paul Gray, speaking from the floor, seconded Smith's suggestion that "the surface that is interesting to the analyst may not be interesting to the patient" (p. 188), although it was not made clear how the two surfaces were defined.

It would seem that the rhetorical voice has once again joined the conversation. So long as "analysts continue to use the term in different ways and contexts associated with different frames of reference" and so long as the "meaning of the surface within the framework of the structural theory remains largely unexplored" (both remarks taken from the introductory comments of the chair; see p. 179), it is difficult to see what good can come of pursuing the discussion, nor does the history of the concept provide any reassurance. *Surface* was initially defined by Freud as referring to what the patient's "unconscious happens to be presenting" (1905), a version that makes particular sense in the context of the then-dominant topographic theory. In subsequent applications, the term has been expanded to mean "the level of observables" (Paniagua, 1985) or the data that can be observed without ambiguity (Paniagua, 1991). Levy and Inderbitzin (1990) extend the concept by making a distinction between the manifest surface, which is the direct observation of the patient's mind, and the latent surface, the level at which the clinician intervenes. Poland (1992) has attempted to enlarge the concept of surface to include the analytic space as well (borrowing the term from Viderman, 1979) and has argued that "the analytic surface can only be appreciated within its context in the analytic space" (p. 385).

A specific example of how this concept has been understood in the everyday clinical encounter is a recent discussion of the analytic surface by Paniagua (1991). As she entered her office one day, she accidentally bumped into a lamp, and the patient (a male) laughed and said, "I do things like that all the time" (p. 679). The analyst describes how she tried to find a way to respond to this comment—to find a thematically similar moment in the subsequent material—and could discover no good opportunity until some four sessions later, when the patient, in talking about a famous sports team and its losing season, admitted that he derived "perverse enjoyment" from their failures (p. 681). We assume that the analyst linked her failure to miss the lamp to the team's losing record. Because it was sufficiently close in meaning to the initial incident, the analyst felt that this remark gave her the opportunity to explore the patient's earlier feelings "with fruitful results in terms of associations and insight" (p. 680). These, unfortunately, are never specified further.

Were there other opportunities? The author admits that "there are always surfaces: the patient's and the clinical ones (fifty minutes of audiovisual surfaces per session)" (p. 680) but claims that she could not find an "adequate workable surface" until the event she describes came to pass. Her remark points up the issue. The study would be considerably enhanced if the author/analyst had found some way to present a fuller sampling of these surfaces to allow the reader to judge whether no other opportunities for intervention had occurred, as she concluded, whether some opportunities had existed that she, for one reason or another, had either not recognized or had chosen not to respond to, and whether the target intervention, when it finally came, was as productive as she claims. As it stands, the report presents only a brief glimpse of a potentially fascinating problem, but without either the full transcript or a fair sample of the intervening hours, we are deprived of the chance to examine the problem of derivatives in more detail. Of particular interest would be those surfaces that seem to the reader to be related to the original incident but were not recognized at the time by the analyst. Her oversight necessarily raises questions about the ways in which local context may disguise meanings and effectively reduce the analyst's sensitivity. The data not presented are undoubtedly rich in implications for the study of different aspects of countertransference.

Although the ambiguity surrounding the word *surface* is never directly addressed, it poses a central problem for understanding Paniagua's thesis. It is not entirely obvious that "material that can be non-conjecturally apperceived by the analyst in the session" (Paniagua's definition of clinical surface; see p. 672) is so easy to define. One suspects that ten analysts would define ten different surfaces (and the panel discussion would seem to support this impression). Here is one place where the presentation of the full transcript seems an essential step toward furthering the discussion. If agreement on "non-conjectural apperception" cannot be found, the concept is already in serious difficulty.

What stands out most clearly in both the summary of the panel discussion and the review of Paniagua's study is that no attempt has been made to reduce the metaphor of analytic surface to something more measurable. The fact that Freud himself used the word *surface* ninety-one times in his writings (see Paniagua, 1991, p. 670) does not justify its continued use in this investigation. One suspects that its metaphoric appeal may be one reason for keeping it in play, yet as we have seen with other rhetorical figures, its very poetic nature interferes with its scientific value. The members of the panel have come under the sway of the rhetorical voice of psychoanalysis. What makes for evocative and persuasive writing does not always make for good science. Before the problem of "surface" can be explored, we need to know more about its ostensive meaning—that is, what the word is pointing at. What are the features of the clinical material that make the analyst choose to respond, and can these features be identified in some reliable and reasonably objective fashion?

A recent study of the analytic surface of one particular case, using a variety of computer-driven methods to look at patterns of speech, provides us with another way of examining the analytic surface. This study had as its goal the search for a specific pattern of words that seemed to trigger an analytic intervention. Because this pattern was not necessarily in the analyst's conscious awareness at the time he was writing up the process notes, it will never be revealed by an anecdotal case report. It was necessary instead to tape-record the six-year analysis; transcribe the tapes, and keypunch the transcripts in order to put the text into a computer-readable format. (Further information about the clinical features of this case—Mrs. C.—and specific findings of the study can be found in Spence, Mayes, and Dahl, in press).

I will present some of the more interesting findings in more detail because the issues they raise are representative of the larger problems faced by the field. In particular, one set of findings would seem to suggest that the analyst is constantly monitoring the clinical material for indications that analyst and analysand are sharing the analytic space. What kind of patterns is he paying attention to? A careful reading of the clinical literature would seem to suggest that the analyst is always scanning the analytic surface in the context of the two-person space, consciously or preconsciously weighing each utterance against the shifting field of connotations provided by the course of the analysis, the history of the analysand's productions, and his own set of associations. When conditions seem favorable, he chooses to enter the analytic space; when conditions are doubtful, he chooses to remain silent. How does he decide?

If it is true that analysts have become more and more concerned with the issue of timing and context, and if it is also true that the content of an interpretation is being increasingly considered within a relational framework, are there certain kinds of language markers that will tell us that *now* is the moment to bring a particular repetition to the patient's attention? In other words, perhaps we can identify both a foreground repetition—the word *failure* in the previous example— and a background repetition that will tell us that the analytic space is safe to enter, that the patient is ready to listen to what we have to say, and/or, in a mood to respond. To search for this kind of window of opportunity is in keeping with the recent emphasis on the "analyst as participant-observer attempting to understand psychic and multiple realities rather than as the arbiter and dispenser of views of objective reality within the analytic situation" (Cooper, 1993, p. 109).

It could be argued that one kind of background signal—one type of invitation to enter the analytic space—may be provided by any indication that both analyst and analysand are, at that moment, sharing the space. How would such sharing be detected? From a series of earlier studies, we came to the conclusion that one way to gauge joint usage of the analytic space would be to monitor the co-occurrence of pronouns marking the two users of that space—*you* and *me*, *you* and *I*, *my* and *yours*, *us* and *we*, and so on. As members of the grammatical class of indexicals, they mark both a spatial location and a temporal moment. Harré (1991) tells us that "the use of the first person in such statements as 'I can feel a draft' labels the content of the utterance with a *spatial location* relative to the location of the speaker and with a *temporal moment* contemporaneous with the event of utterance" (p. 59). By the same reasoning, the co-occurrence of *you* and *me*, spoken by a patient on the couch, marks off both a spatial location (she is talking to us) and a temporal moment—a moment, we can argue, that can be seen as a window of opportunity for an intervention.

If the words *you* and *me* co-occur equally often in the patient's discourse, we have reason to believe that she is jointly considering the analyst and herself in her thoughts, fantasies, and plans. It stands to reason that an intervention at this particular moment would have a greater likelihood of being heard and understood than an intervention at some other time (for example, when only first person or third person pronouns are being used). This line of reasoning allows us to use the co-occurrence rate of pronouns such as *you/me* as a measure of a shared analytic space. In successful cases, we would expect that the analyst would tend to intervene when this measure is high and fall silent when it is low. The co-occurrence rate should thus be positively correlated with the number of interventions.

Obviously, counting pronouns is not the way most analysts spend their time with patients, and it would be foolish to expect that any analyst could give a reasonable estimate of the frequency of the pronouns *you* and *me* in an analytic hour. (If he could actually come within 25 percent of the correct figure, we might worry about his clinical work). But earlier research on subliminal stimuli (see Spence and Holland, 1962) and the use of certain kinds of marker words by cancer patients (Spence, Scarborough, and Ginsberg, 1978) has convinced us of our remarkable sensitivity to minor variations in the language. These data would argue that it was quite possible for the analyst to *preconsciously* sense variations in the co-occurrence of certain pronouns, and that this awareness might easily bias his decision about when to make an intervention. It is also possible that the important markers may have been uttered with slightly different vocal inflections, and although we have no data on this point, it suggests an interesting line of investigation for the future.

If *you* and *me* are markers of time and place, it should also follow that the extent of their separation in the patient's discourse might give us some sense of the strength of the alliance between patient and analyst. A single *you* followed many sentences later by a single *me* (high separation) is telling quite a different story than a pair of pronouns separated by only a few words (low separation). Median separation should be negatively correlated with a shared analytic surface and, therefore, with number of interventions. The degree of separation we will call SEPtrans, which stands for the median separation of pairs of pronouns marking the transference. Co-occurrence rate we will call CORtrans, which is the number of pairs of co-occurring pronouns, such as *you/me,* divided by the total words uttered.

How do these variables behave in a clinical setting? Suppose a new patient is beginning her treatment and she asks, from the couch, "What do you want me to call you?" Here is an example of two co-occurrences: *you/me* and *me/you*—with a median separation of 2.5 words. Dividing the number by the total number of words (8) gives us a rate of .25. Suppose, on the other hand, that she says, "I think

I'll use the title Silent One during this ordeal." The co-occurrence rate is 0 and the median separation is 0. (Both the co-occurrence rates and separation scores tend to reflect the intimacy of the exchange.)

There are other times when the patient is talking and we feel that we are really not in the room. We might guess that these sessions would show a minimal number of *you/me* co-occurrences and a high degree of separation. At the same time, the patient's discourse might show a high number of *I/me* co-occurrences, and we developed a separate score to measure pairings that refer to different aspects of the patient's self. Making any kind of intervention under these conditions is a little bit like taking part in a conference call—the analyst's voice is one of many, simply being added to the *I/me* conversation already taking place inside the patient's head.

Seventy analytic hours were selected from the well-studied case of Mrs. C.—a successful, six-year analysis that has been investigated by many research teams over the past twenty years. The patient, a married social worker in her late twenties, had sought treatment because of lack of sexual responsiveness, difficulty in experiencing pleasurable feelings, and low self-esteem. She was the second of four children from a professional family. She was seen five times a week. (Further details about this case can be found in Jones and Windholz, 1990.)

The hours in question cover all six years of the case. In addition to being computer-ready, they had all been rated by Enrico Jones and his team from Berkeley using a list of one hundred clinical items called the Psychotherapy Process Q-Sort (described in Jones and Windholz, 1990). This list contains three types of items: those describing patient attitudes and behavior or experience; those reflecting therapist actions and attitudes; and those attempting to capture the nature of the interaction of the dyad, the climate or atmosphere of the encounter. Among the first group were such items as "Patient relies upon therapist to solve his/her problems"; among the second were such items as "Therapist condescends to, or patronizes the patient," or "Therapist is tactless"; and among the third, "There is an erotic quality to the therapy relationship."

One of the features of this case that made it ideal for our purposes was that it was conducted by a classical analyst who believed in making minimal interventions. The number varied from 2 to 25 per session with a mean of 9. This feature of the case was crucial to our plans, because with relatively few interventions in each hour, we were able to relate their appearance to changes in our two measures of pronoun use. Had there been more frequent interventions, the task would have been much more difficult, if not impossible.

The seventy hours were divided into seven blocks of ten hours each. Two blocks were taken from the first year of treatment, and all subsequent blocks from subsequent years. Each block consisted of ten contiguous hours. All seventy hours were scored for number of interventions and (by computer) for frequency and median separation of pairs of shared pronouns such as *you/me, me/you, you/I, I/you,* and so on. To determine frequency, we counted the number of times the first word of any pair was followed by the second within a search space of a thousand characters or less; the total number of pairs found per analytic hour was divided by the number of words spoken. To determine separation, we looked at the distribution of all pairs of pronouns and computed the median distance of this set of scores.

The correlation between frequency of co-occurring pronouns and number of interventions is significant ($r = .30$, $p = .01$). When co-occurrence rate is high, the analyst tends to intervene; when it is low, he remains silent. It would appear that he pays attention (probably at a preconscious level) to the co-occurrence rate of shared pairs of pronouns as he monitors the analytic surface and uses this rate to determine when he should make an intervention. When we look at this relationship over time, we find that it becomes increasingly positive as the analysis progresses, and in a final block of ten hours, the correlation reaches a high of .82 ($p < .01$), suggesting that when this phase of treatment is reached, the analyst seems to be using pronoun co-occurrence as one of the primary methods of determining when to enter the analytic space.

In order to understand this finding in more detail, we divided each of the hours in the last block (Nos. 936–945) into equal-sized segments of approximately five hundred words each and scored each segment for frequency, separation, and number of interventions. The correlation increases in significance ($p < .005$, 82 d.f.) with an increase in data points, and a graph of the function shows that the analyst's interventions tend to closely track the co-occurrence rate of shared pairs of pronouns.

Median separation is not related to number of interventions across the full set of seventy hours, but a relationship did emerge in the fine-grained analysis of the last ten hours ($r = -.29$, $p < .01$). The negative correlation would suggest that interventions increase as median distance decreases; in other words, the analyst monitors the analytic space not only with respect to frequency, but also with respect to the distance, in the patient's discourse, between members of such pronoun pairs as *you/me*. If these pairs are spaced far apart, he tends to remain quiet; if they cluster close together (within the same sentence, for example), he will tend to make an intervention.

These data add a new dimension to the concept of analytic surface. It would appear that at the same time the analyst in the session is responding to problems of drive and defense, transference and countertransference, he is also responding to subtle changes in the patterning of the patient's speech that tell him when it is safe (and fruitful) to enter the analytic space. While he is almost certainly consciously unaware of specific changes in pronoun frequency or location, the lawfulness of their connection to the analyst's activity would indicate that at a preconscious level, he is responding to subtle changes in the clinical material. The data also make us aware that it may be necessary to distinguish between *manifest* and *latent* triggers of an intervention. What the analyst believes to be the reason for entering the analytic space—the manifest cause—may be quite different from the actual trigger, a change in speech pattern, which acts as the latent cause. Many of our technical rules of thumb may turn out, on closer examination, to contain only part of the truth, and will need to be revised in the light of future research.

These data also have implications for the case study problem. If timing proves to be as important a variable as they suggest, we need to think carefully about the best method of recording our clinical material. Not only does the traditional case study format make it difficult, if not impossible, to measure the distance (in minutes and seconds) from the onset of a particular intervention to a particular pattern in the clinical material, it also tends to focus our attention on the purely lexical meaning of the interpretation rather than on its place in the analytic conversation. The traditional method also tends to focus attention on interventions deemed important by the analyst, and not to report other parts of the interchange (such as pronoun distribution) that may be of equal or greater significance. And whatever is reported tends to be reported anecdotally and not veridically, giving us the sense of what was said but rarely, if ever, its exact meaning. New methods of data collection need to be developed that will capture such important variables as point of onset and change in contingent responsiveness over time, and enable us to begin to investigate the intricate structure of the patient-analyst dialogue. None of these variables can be determined from the usual kind of anecdotal case presentation.

Computer-guided content analysis of the analytic surface can also uncover other kinds of regularities that are probably not in the analyst's conscious awareness at the time he is conducting the case or writing up his report. It turns out that this patient, Mrs. C., showed a particular fondness for the expression "you know"; it appeared in forty-three of the seventy hours studied, with an overall frequency ranging from 0 to 93 (and a mean frequency of 12 per session). It has the additional significance of being highly correlated with certain kinds of interventions. For example, when the analyst points out the use of defensive maneuvers, the frequency of this marker tends to increase ($r = .74$, $p < .001$). By the same token, when the analyst identifies a recurrent theme in the patient's experience or when termination is discussed, the frequency of *you know* also tends to increase ($r = .66$; $r = .71$; both correlations significant at $p < .001$). On the other hand, it is not correlated with number of interventions ($r = .14$, n.s.).

When we compare the two types of response measures in the speech of Mrs. C., it would seem to follow that we can make a distinction between *derivatives* and *openings*. The expression "you know" appears to accompany a somewhat heightened emotional state and seems to be triggered by the specific types of interpretations listed above. It can be understood as a kind of linguistic buffer, a pausing device that allowed her to prepare to say something more forceful than was her custom. It often preceded an expression of strong affect. If the thoughts and feelings being aroused were more than usually conflicted, it is not surprising that the number of *you know*'s would increase.

This marker, however, is not triggered by just any intervention; as we have seen, the correlation with all interventions is only .14. Co-occurring shared pronouns, on the other hand, are correlated with all interventions. We can think of the first type of marker as being a direct consequence of specific meanings—a classical derivative—whereas the second type can be thought of, not as the result of an intervention, but rather, as a signal that an intervention can now be introduced. It announces an opening in the analytic surface. We see now that one set of correlations—those associated with derivatives—signals the impact of the analyst's remarks on the patient's speech, whereas the other set of correlations marks the reverse: the moments in the clinical material that trigger the analyst's response.

Toward the end of her paper on the analytic surface, Paniagua admits that "at our present state of knowledge, the definition of workable surface cannot be specific, since we seem to lack consistent data to be able to objectify it reliably" (1991, pp. 679–680). It would seem that one step toward this highly necessary objectification is the accumulation of a large number of completely transcribed, computer-readable analytic cases that could be searched for derivatives and openings in an attempt to establish both reliability and generality. Where Paniagua believes that the level of observables lies at the level of the clinical surface (p. 682), it is becoming apparent that this surface is composed of a wide variety of markers, some readily available to the experienced analyst, others somewhat more disguised, and still others waiting to be discovered.

Only the careful study of a wide range of cases conducted by a broad spectrum of analysts will allow us to discover the more important aspects of this surface and how they are related to analytic work. For example, it seems more than likely that derivatives may be more easily identified than openings, if only because we tend to listen for specific reactions after making an interpretation (and because it is easier to keep track of a fixed pair of words, such as *you know,* than to listen for a co-occurring pair separated by varying amounts of intervening language). It also seems likely that a certain number of technical difficulties may stem from the confusion of one category with another. When Paniagua was describing her search for the proper moment to respond to her patient, she was probably looking for the appropriate opening, and her need to wait for four sessions may be an indication that the opening was subtle and hard to discover. But because the derivatives are more obvious, it may sometimes be tempting to use them to trigger an intervention, although such a move may be mistaken because they are not necessarily a reliable point of entry into the analytic space. One kind of clinical wisdom can probably be described as the knowledge *not* to respond at seemingly obvious moments (derivatives) and to wait instead for more subtle indicators (openings).

The findings also have implications for the measurement of free-floating attention. One way to explain the high correlation between co-occurrence frequency and interventions in the last ten hours of the case is to assume that the analyst was becoming more skilled at adopting the modal analytic stance of free-floating attention and was, as a result, becoming more sensitive to such subtle indicators as pronoun pairings. Spencer and Balter (1990) have argued that when the analyst is taking full advantage of the analyzing instrument, he is more likely to be influenced by primary process aspects of the clinical material: "acoustic images, displacement, and contiguity" (p. 414). We would include the contiguity of shared pronouns in this category and make the argument that the analyst's increasing sensitivity to this marker over the life of the case of Mrs. C. would suggest that he had entered into a more regressive mode of listening. It follows that high correlations between co-occurrence and number of interventions might be used as one criterion for having entered this mode.

Escaping the Rhetorical Voice

Terms such as *surface* or *depth* or *analytic space* tend to be evocative, even comforting, in their metaphoric promise but almost always turn out to be unreliable in practice because connotation tends to displace denotation. Paniagua is entirely right in pointing out that the concept of *surface* has never been reliably defined, but she does not seem to realize that this step can never be taken until we can agree on new rules of evidence and new standards of presentation. One of the lessons to be drawn from the preceding chapters is that psychoanalysis has failed to convert metaphor into anything like responsible science. It has, as we have repeatedly seen, taken refuge in rhetoric as a final explanation. (In his opening remarks to the panel discussion on analytic surface, Inderbitzin "asked the panelists to join in a Freudian spirit of inquiry—to follow out this idea of the analytic surface, if for no other reason than the pleasure of seeing where it will take us"; see Seelig, 1993, p. 180.) It has depended on argument by authority in contrast to what Habermas (1971) has called the "dialogue of uncompelled consensus." It has failed to find a language that adequately represents things like wishes and fantasies, which are psychically real but objectively invisible. After the initial success of Freud's more arresting metaphors, it became clear that their referents would be forever out of reach and that metaphoric description was little different from Wittgenstein's private language and subject to all its faults. Poetry is not the same as pointing.

Second, the classical approach has been unable to give up its fascination with Freud and move on to other thinkers and other observations. Repeated references to Freud are not the same as a growing body of replicated findings, and it may be this fascination with its founder that has prevented psychoanalysis from abandoning the traditional case study format and experimenting with some new mode of presentation.

Third, the classical approach has been unable to find an answer to the problem of secrecy and privileged access. Only a minority of essential information is in the public domain, and much of this has been so disguised, for reasons of confidentiality, that its reliability must be called into question. In contrast to the practices of other disciplines, the lion's share of our clinical wisdom, as we have seen, is stored in the minds of practitioners and in this somewhat transient state is simply not accessible to any attempts at validation. Because we have no public archive of clinical happenings that is open to inspection by any interested party, our "data," largely stored as memories, are all the time being shaped by whatever theory is most popular. And because the "data" are largely illusory, we have no chance to build theory in the usual way, from the bottom up. Psychoanalysis is a top-down science, pure and simple. With no data to contradict them, theories tend to take over, and their rhetorical voice—and not their content—plays a large role in their persuasive appeal. (The very sensitivity to rhetoric that made possible this observation is, of course, one of the contributions of the hermeneutic left).

Fourth, the heavy hand of theory has all but eliminated research from the psychoanalytic enterprise. The few studies that are published are either "impeccably scientific studies of nothing very much, or . . . exciting but cloudy psychoanalytic speculations" (Dinnage, 1991, p. 7). Research findings we have every reason to believe (because they come from studies whose methodology is flawless) unfortunately tend to be unrelated to issues of clinical significance or relevance. But the more interesting, even exciting clinical studies are flawed by their reliance on anecdote, their failure to collect a complete set of data, their untroubled reliance on metaphor and other rhetorical devices, and last of all—and perhaps most important—by a medieval belief in the idea that what is sensed by one investigator must be seen by all. Whereas children of five or six have usually become aware of the fact that their thoughts may be different from those of their peers or their elders (see Astington, Harris, and Olson, 1988), this possibility seems to have escaped most analytic researchers. As a result, there is no provision for the play of subjectivity in the evaluation of evidence, no sign that the researcher needs to guard against unwitting bias or the confounding effect of theory on observation.

Fifth, the classical approach has been unable to find a home for what has been called the Roshomon effect—the fact that almost anything worth looking at has at least two sides to it. It still pretends that psychoanalysis, sooner or later, will take the form of normal science and rule complications of individual differences out of order. And yet it is problems of subjectivity that we meet every day in both our patients and ourselves, and it is one of the arguments of the hermeneutic left that construal of meanings is always a personal adventure, framed by the context of the moment, and that this context can never be perfectly translated or exported. Our clinical observations are *always* colored by our private context. Subjectivity not only affects the patient's view of the transference, it influences the beginning candidate's report to his supervisor and the senior analyst's write-up of his case as well as his memory of his most recent interpretation and his view of the state of the profession.

Why has it been so difficult to give up the rhetorical voice? One reason why rhetoric reigns supreme is that psychoanalysis has never found a way to represent its most important data in some form of shareable, unambiguous language. It has always seemed preferable to adopt poetic language wherever possible, not only because of Freud's example, but also because metaphors and similar figures have an almost mythological appeal. They also tend to satisfy a wide range of practitioners because, as we have seen, these terms fit directly into our private thoughts about our patients and because their very vagueness seems to promise agreement. More narrowly defined denotative or ostensive terms may not always seem to fit the occasion. And yet, as Paniagua's paper makes clear, to stay at the level of such terms as the *analytic surface* is to remain forever rooted in a metaphor that promises much but delivers next to nothing. Arguments carried out at this level supported by data gathered in the anecdotal tradition could easily continue for decades or even centuries without affecting either our permanent store of knowledge or the opinions of any of the debaters.

How exactly can we define the optimal *evidential surface* for analytic investigation? A quick glance through a recent issue of any
journal shows an unspoken agreement that the data of significance
can be framed in such terms as *surface, depth, empathy, transference,
analytic process, enactment,* and similar language from our shared
clinical vocabulary. As I have noted, language of this kind is used all
the time in our clinical work and in framing problems of strategy and
tactics in our approach to patients. The profession has not yet developed a vocabulary that might link this largely figurative language to
specific aspects of the clinical material. Our analysis of specific hours
from the case of Mrs. C. has made clear the fact that the analytic
surface can be divided into at least two dimensions—derivatives and
openings—and further research would undoubtedly extend this list.
But this discovery can only be made when we move from the evidential
surface of the usual case report to a more fine-grained analysis of the
clinical transcript, an analysis that is supplemented by computer—an
important and perhaps essential next step. It never would have happened if we remained at the conventional anecdotal level.

Our analysis of Mrs. C. also revealed the not-so-surprising fact that
there is a lawfulness in the analyst's behavior that operates below the
level of conscious awareness and can therefore only be discovered by
moving beyond self-report. The profession has always prided itself on
its superior sensitivity to subjective experience and has relied on this
skill to explore and clarify many kinds of clinical encounters. But there
are clearly limits to this sensitivity, and no amount of analytic training
or self-analysis could ever enable an analyst to be able to reliably
monitor his awareness of such subtle cues as pronoun pairing or pronoun separation. It follows that these kinds of variables will never be
discovered if we continue to define the evidential surface as it is currently described in our major journals and, most recently, in a panel
on its uses (Seelig, 1993).

What is more, our justified respect for introspection and insight can
often blind us to the fact that self-knowledge is often unreliable and
misleading. If the evidential surface is taken to be the equivalent of
our normal clinical awareness, we are always at the mercy of countertransference intrusions, and to date, the profession has found no
way of policing this kind of contamination and excluding its influence
from our published case reports. We are also at the mercy of the writer's gift for language. Because there is no standard, shareable method
of introspection, we depend on a sensitivity to phrasing that not all

authors are capable of; as a result, our access to the shared evidential surface is highly variable, and while some reports are little master-pieces of insight, others, because of their wooden language or inept phrasing, are uninformative and perhaps even misleading.

Another reason for moving to a different evidential surface in our publications has to do with the issue I discussed in Chapter 8—the fact that many of the so-called "discoveries" made by this or that theorist are frequently no more than "projections" of the theorist's own private history. We would appear to have a kind of double stan-dard with regard to psychological relativism. We appreciate how our patients can misunderstand our deliberately composed analytic neu-trality and project onto our utterances any number of extraneous—and sometimes outrageous—readings; this kind of distortion is seen every day in our clinical work, and working through these distortions represents a large part of our analytic activity. But the problem takes on quite a different shape when interpretations surface in a theoretical context, even though the underlying phenomenon remains the same. For someone like Rangell (1991), castration anxiety is a self-evident and demonstrable fact, to be seen at every turn in the average clinical practice; failure to see it counts as an obvious error. For a Kleinian, the facts of childhood observation should force us to conclude that the child very early comes to realize that the mother can be dangerous, even evil, and that failure to agree can only be classed as an almost criminal form of oversight. For the classical analyst, the oedipal tri-angle is a fact of life, and any attempt to claim otherwise can only be seen as impertinent, argumentative, and above all, unnecessary. But is not each of these positions an example of theoretical relativism that parallels the kind of tunnel vision (and sometimes, the use of projec-tion and identification) that we see all the time in our patients? An agreement on a new kind of evidential surface would help to protect against some of these influences. It can be seen that if a fine-grained look at other analyses shows a correlation between interventions and pronoun co-occurrences similar to what was found with Mrs. C., the personal history of the investigator becomes less of a contaminating factor.

In making the argument that the field has to move to a new eviden-tial surface if it is to make any respectable advance in the next ten or twenty years, I am taking issue with Wallerstein and his comforting overview of the relation of theory to data. Where he concludes that clinical facts are "anchored directly enough to observables, to the data of the consulting room" (1988, p. 17) that the testing and validation of theory follows the standard procedures of normal science, I would call this belief into question. As we have seen with the example of analytic surface—and any number of other problematic concepts could be put in its place—the term only pretends to be denotative in its reference. In fact, the definition of analytic surface varies with the definer, and the so-called surface is probably composed of any number of clinical events that function in different ways and have varying degrees of information value for the analyst. Some (what we have labeled openings) appear to be invitations to enter the analytic space; others (so-called derivatives) appear to be the consequences of specific interventions perhaps better listened to in silence. Other clinical moments remain to be identified. But so long as the dialogue remains at the level of the analytic surface or the workable surface (to use Paniagua's more recent formulation), we will never discover these more specific ingredients.

10 Two Kinds of Knowing

In the concluding section of a chapter on quantitative research in psychoanalysis, Luborsky and I summed up our review with the observation that "psychoanalysts, like other psychotherapists, literally *do not know* how they achieve their results, although they have searched longer and deeper than others and possess a unique store of clinical wisdom. They have learned their craft from a long line of practitioners schooled in a master-apprentice relationship; the rules are taught more by example than by explanation" (1979, pp. 360–361).

Although true from within one frame of reference, this conclusion does not tell the whole story. It might be more accurate to say that analysts do indeed know how they make successful interpretations and bring about cures, but the knowing in question does not refer to rational knowledge but to something closer to *gnosis,* or reflective knowing. The difference between scientific and reflective knowledge is captured in the distinction in French between *savoir* and *connaître,* in German between *kennen* and *wissen,* and in English between *knowledge* and *wisdom* (Pagels, 1979, p. xix, and personal communication). It is the difference between knowing *that* and knowing *about,* and the history of psychoanalysis has been the story of how we can translate one form of knowing into the other. *Gnosis* is a perfectly useful form of knowledge for the individual analyst who is practicing his craft and treating his patient, but it does not travel well at professional meetings or across publications because it is based on a mixture of theory and private language seasoned with a sprinkling of body wisdom, some vague memories of clinical moments, and perhaps a mixture of other sensations aroused by the ambience of the consulting room, the rhythm of the analysand's voice, the way the afternoon sunlight strikes the window in late spring, and a host of other stimuli, some of which he is aware of and some not. Some of this mixture can be distilled into such well-worn concepts as *analytic surface* or *psychic structure,* which can then be exchanged at meetings and argued over in discussion groups, but this does not solve the problem. The notion of *analytic surface* reflects a collective wisdom that has been accumulating since the beginning of psychoanalysis, but since each analyst defines it in his own way, it still remains *gnosis,* not practical knowledge.

In Chapter 9 we saw that it is possible to isolate one aspect of the analytic surface—pronoun co-occurrence—and both measure it reliably and relate it to such other dimensions as frequency of interventions and content of interpretation. The chapter described the move from wisdom to knowledge—from knowing (imprecisely) *when* to make an intervention to knowing (more exactly) *why* we make it (in the case of Mrs. C.) at a particular moment. But we need to realize that other aspects of the analytic surface are going to be much more resistant to this kind of translation because they are based on variables that we still have no way of measuring (such as the analyst's context of consciousness at a particular moment or the clinical impressions left by previous patients). Context is important in part because it changes the meaning of the clinical happening at that particular moment, and this line of reasoning brings us back to the importance of the specimen in all its depth of detail.

The importance of the moment puts the burden of discovery back onto the practicing clinician. We must appeal to him to turn wisdom into knowledge by providing us with fruitful metaphors and other figures of speech that will turn the multiple sensations of the clinical moment into transparent language accessible to all. We can think of the field of psychoanalytic knowledge (in company with other fields of science) as a "man-made fabric which impinges on experience only along the edges. Or, to change the figure, total science is like a field of force whose boundary conditions are experience" (Quine, 1953, p. 78). Once we move away from the edges, Quine continues, the total field of knowledge is so "underdetermined by its boundary conditions, experience, that there is much latitude of choice as to what statements to reevaluate in the light of any single contrary experience." A new understanding of the evidential surface *might* have a significant influence on those concepts that are close to the edge of experience, but it would not affect terms farther away. For large parts of our conceptual network that do not impinge on experience, there is almost no limit to the ways in which we can formulate our clinical activity. In this Alice-in-Wonderland state of affairs, all voices are equal—but all run the risk of being equally wrong. And because our concepts are largely unrelated to the hard edge of reality, they can be argued over indefinitely. Fashion and rhetorical appeal become the arbiters of taste. Psychoanalytic politics elbows science aside. But knowledge does not accumulate.

Once we define the analytic surface in terms of pronoun co-occurrence, we begin to link a conceptual term to a repeatable observation. Other parts of the analytic surface remain somewhat more removed from the boundary that "impinges on experience," and it is here that we need the advice of the practicing analyst to provide us with ways of going from reflective knowledge to practical knowledge. But since it is perfectly possible to practice analytic work in isolation entirely on the basis of *gnosis,* there is no compelling reason to assume the burden of translation unless the profession at large begins to feel dissatisfied with the old ways of knowing.

In the latter days of the Ptolemaic theory, more and more accurate observations of planets and stars made it increasingly obvious that they did not revolve around the earth in simple circles as the theory would predict. To account for the precession of the equinoxes, it was necessary to assume that each planet revolved in a small circle, or epicycle, as it was tracing its larger orbit around the earth. But observation continued to violate theory, and it was necessary to add more and more epicycles and make their orbits increasingly eccentric. But finally, of course, even this patchwork system failed to match experience "along the edges," and it was replaced by the Copernican theory in which the sun, not the earth, became the center of the solar system. All of a sudden, epicycles were no longer needed and computations became almost trivial.

Dissatisfaction with badly fitting theory may encourage some analysts to close the gap between theory and observation, but the uneasiness necessary for this move is far from being epidemic at the moment. As I pointed out in the first chapter, it is still possible to find specific circumstances that seem to conform to a Ptolemaic, geocentric model. There are many boundary conditions that are not disconfirmed by outdated theories. There are many clinical accounts that seem to support Freud's oedipal formulation or a vague concept of the analytic surface. A romantic astronomer, fixated in the past, could easily fill up his life by taking observations of the time and place of sunrise and sunset, and nothing in his data would contradict the thesis that the earth was the center of the universe. In similar fashion, a self-satisfied psychoanalyst can still find a good fit between standard theory and the memory of his latest analytic hour. He can still find pockets that seem to support outmoded theory or reinforce the use of ambiguous metaphor. But data collection of this kind is not true science because it turns a blind eye on all those occasions, past and present, when theory is not supported by the data. Spirits may be lifted by these observations but science suffers because by holding on to old dogma or by inventing new epicycles, we miss the true beauty, majesty, and lawfulness of the clinical encounter. The enterprise Freud began with such promise ends up being fascinated with its own reflection—and seeing nothing else.

Thus the struggle between knowledge and wisdom is a struggle over whether history is sacred and meant to be slavishly followed or whether it is to be seen more as something onto which we can climb (the well-known shoulders of giants) to make ever greater discoveries. As the Copernican theory made it clear that epicycles were no longer needed in everyday computations of planetary positions, its very elegance became part of its appeal. Perhaps something similar will happen with psychoanalytic theory, because as our knowledge of key concepts (such as analytic surface) becomes more refined, it becomes more clinically useful, leading to better-timed interventions and, eventually, to more effective treatments. As the marketplace of ideas begins to prefer knowledge over wisdom, other parts of the analytic surface will be reformulated and made more accessible. As our language becomes more precise, we can begin to move farther and farther from the edge of experience. Slowly, very slowly, knowledge will begin to take over from wisdom.

Yet here I would mention three cautions. It would be a mistake, as I noted in Chapter 7, to move too quickly from specific observation to general law; we should guard against the temptation to become a "real" science overnight. Before observations become laws, we need, first, to expand our net of clinical observations and, second, to find a new language that will mediate between clinical metaphor and analytic theory. Forming laws prematurely will not only preempt our search for an intervening language, it will tend to overlook critical differences between clinical happenings.

A second caution bears on the mediating language. It must be responsive not only to the data of observation—the clinical happening—but in addition, to the analyst's context of consciousness. If, for example, the analyst is about to leave on vacation, he will tend to hear all references to interruptions and journeys as pertaining to him; his context of consciousness will necessarily "harmonize" the patient's discourse with his particular background concerns. Some way must be found to provide the reader with both melody and accompaniment and enable him to "hear" the patient's utterances as the analyst did.

Finally, ways must be found to share the working knowledge—the "folk psychology"—of practicing analysts, and to take steps to avoid burying individual differences under standard terminology. One of the problems with concepts such as analytic surface is that they override the individual analyst's highly specific understanding; a too quick recourse to standard terms risks the disappearance of hard-won experience, and as I noted in Chapter 1, this experience is stored largely in the minds of living practitioners. It is by savoring the detail that we can best move from wisdom to knowledge, and an effort must be made to capture the detail before it gets lost.

References
Index

References

Astington, J. W., P. L. Harris, and D. R. Olson. 1988. *Developing Theories of Mind*. Cambridge: Cambridge Univ. Press.

Balter, L., Z. Lothane, and J. H. Spencer. 1980. On the analyzing instrument. *Psychoanalytic Quarterly*, 49: 474–504.

Bernstein, R. J. 1983. *Beyond Objectivism and Relativism*. Philadelphia: Univ. of Pennsylvania Press.

Bettelheim, B. 1983. *Freud and Man's Soul*. New York: Knopf.

Blight, J. 1981. Must psychoanalysis retreat to hermeneutics? Psychoanalytic theory in the light of Popper's evolutionary epistemology. *Psychoanalysis and Contemporary Thought*, 4: 147–205.

Bonaparte, M., A. Freud, and E. Kris (Eds.). 1954. *The Origins of Psychoanalysis*. New York: Basic Books.

Bowie, M. 1988. *Freud, Proust and Lacan: Theory as Fiction*. Cambridge: Cambridge Univ. Press.

Boyd, R. 1979. Metaphor and theory change: What is 'Metaphor' a Metaphor For? In A. Ortony (Ed.), *Metaphor and Thought*. Cambridge: Cambridge Univ. Press, pp. 356–408.

Brenner, C. 1982. *The Mind in Conflict*. New York: International Universities Press.

Brenner, C. 1985. Book review of Merton Gill's *Analysis of Transference*. *Journal of the American Psychoanalytic Association*, 33: 241–244.

Broyard, A. 1989. Does your analyst read Henry James? *New York Times Book Review*, April 16, 1989, pp. 14–15.

Bruner, J. 1986. *Actual Minds, Possible Worlds*. Cambridge, Mass.: Harvard Univ. Press.

Bylebyl, J. J. 1985. Disputation and description in the Renaissance pulse controversy. In Wear et al., pp. 223–245.

Campbell, D. T. 1986. Science's social system of validity-enhancing collective belief change and the problems of social sciences. In D. W. Fiske and R. A. Shweder (Eds.), *Metatheory in Social Science*. Chicago: Univ. of Chicago Press.

Cavell, M. 1988. Solipsism and community. *Psychoanalysis and Contemporary Thought,* 11: 587–613.

Clark, R. 1980. *Freud: The Man and the Cause*. New York: Random House.

Cooper, S. H. 1993. Interpretive fallibility and the psychoanalytic dialogue. *Journal of the American Psychoanalytic Association,* 41: 95–126.

Crews, F. 1988. Beyond Sulloway's *Freud:* Psychoanalysis minus the myth of the hero. In P. Clark and C. Wright (Eds.), *Mind, Psychoanalysis and Science*. Oxford: Basil Blackwell.

Crombie, A. C. 1979. *Augustine to Galileo,* vols. 1 and 2. Cambridge, Mass.: Harvard Univ. Press.

Cuddon, J. A. 1977. *A Dictionary of Literary Terms*. New York: Doubleday.

Cunningham, A. 1985. Fabricus and the "Aristotle project" in anatomical teaching and research at Padua. In Wear et al., pp. 195–222.

Dahl, H., V. Teller, D. Moss, and M. Trujillo. 1978. Countertransference examples of the syntactic expression of warded-off contents. *Psychoanalytic Quarterly,* 47: 339–363.

Darwin, C. 1890. *The Voyage of the Beagle*. New York: Appleton.

Davidson, D. 1980. Mental events. In *Actions and Events*. Oxford: Oxford Univ. Press.

Davies, R. 1970. *Fifth Business*. New York: Penguin Books.

Debus, A. G. 1965. *The English Paracelsians*. New York: Franklin Watts.

Dinnage, R. 1991. The wounded male. *Times Literary Supplement,* December 13, p. 7.

Eissler, K. R. 1971. *Talent and Genius: The Fictitious Case of Tausk Contra Freud*. New York: Quadrangle Books.

Ellenberger, H. 1970. *The Discovery of the Unconscious: History and Evolution of Dynamic Psychiatry*. New York: Basic Books.

Ellmann, R., and C. Feidelson. 1965. *The Modern Tradition*. New York: Oxford Univ. Press.

Emde, R. N. 1992. Individual meaning and increasing complexity: Contributions of Sigmund Freud and Rene Spitz to developmental psychology. *Developmental Psychology,* 28: 347–359.

Felman, S. 1983. Beyond Oedipus: The specimen story of psychoanalysis. *Modern Language Notes,* 95: 1021–1053.

Fiedler, L. 1966. *Love and Death in the American Novel*. New York: Stein and Day.

Firth, R. 1936. *We, the Tikopia*. London: Allen & Unwin.

Fish, S. 1986. Withholding the missing portion: Power, meaning and persuasion in Freud's "The Wolf Man." *Times Literary Supplement,* August 29, pp. 935–938.

Fisher, S., and R. P. Greenberg. 1977. *The Scientific Credibility of Freud's Theories and Therapy.* New York: Basic Books.

Flexner, A. 1910. *Medical Education in the United States and Canada.* New York: Carnegie Foundation for the Advancement of Teaching.

Foucault, M. 1973. *The Order of Things.* New York: Vintage Books.

Freud, S. 1896. The Aetiology of hysteria. *Standard Edition,* vol. 3. London: Hogarth Press.

Freud, S. 1900. Die Traumdeutung. *Standard Edition,* vols. 4 & 5. London: Hogarth Press.

Freud, S. 1905. Fragments of an analysis of a case of hysteria. *Standard Edition,* vol. 7. London: Hogarth Press.

Freud, S. 1909. Notes upon a case of obsessional neurosis. *Standard Edition,* vol. 10. London: Hogarth Press.

Freud, S. 1912. Recommendations to physicians practicing psycho-analysis. *Standard Edition,* vol. 12. London: Hogarth Press.

Freud, S. 1913. On beginning the treatment. *Standard Edition,* vol. 12. London: Hogarth Press.

Freud, S. 1914. On narcissism: An introduction. *Standard Edition,* vol. 14. London: Hogarth Press.

Freud, S. 1915. Instincts and their vicissitudes. *Standard Edition,* vol. 14. London: Hogarth Press.

Freud, S. 1916. Introductory Lectures on Psycho-analysis, I–II. *Standard Edition,* vol. 15. London: Hogarth Press.

Freud, S. 1918. From the history of an infantile neurosis. *Standard Edition,* vol. 17. London: Hogarth Press.

Freud, S. 1920. Beyond the pleasure principle. *Standard Edition,* vol. 18. London: Hogarth Press.

Freud. S. 1925. An autobiographical study. *Standard Edition,* vol. 20. London: Hogarth Press.

Freud, S. 1933. New introductory lectures on psycho-analysis. *Standard Edition,* vol. 22. London: Hogarth Press.

Freud, S. 1937. Constructions in analysis. *Standard Edition,* vol. 23. London: Hogarth Press.

Fussell, P. 1975. *The Great War and Modern Memory.* New York: Oxford Univ. Press.

Gardner, H. 1983. *Frames of Mind.* New York: Basic Books.

Garrison, P. 1991. *Augury.* Athens: Univ. of Georgia Press.

Gay, P. 1988. *Freud: A Life for Our Time.* New York: W. W. Norton.

Geertz, C. 1988. *Works and Lives: The Anthropologist as Author*. Stanford: Stanford Univ. Press.

Gergen, K. J. 1985. The social constructionist movement in modern psychology. *American Psychologist,* 40: 266–275.

Gergen, K. J., and M. Gergen. 1986. Narrative form and the construction of psychological science. In T. R. Sarbin (Ed.), *Narrative Psychology*. New York: Praeger.

Goldberg, A. (Ed.). 1978. *The Psychology of the Self: A Casebook*. New York: International Universities Press.

Greenwald, A. G., A. R. Pratkanis, M. R. Leippe, and M. H. Baumgardner. 1986. Under what conditions does theory obstruct research progress? *Psychological Review,* 93: 216–229.

Grinstein, A. 1983. *Freud's Rules of Dream Interpretation*. New York: International Universities Press.

Grossman, W. I., and B. Simon. 1969. Anthropomorphism: Motive, meaning and causality in psychoanalytic theory. *Psychoanalytic Study of the Child,* 24: 78–111.

Grünbaum, A. 1984. *The Foundations of Psychoanalysis*. Berkeley: Univ. of California Press.

Grünbaum, A. 1988. The role of the case study method in the foundations of psychoanalysis. *Canadian Journal of Philosophy,* 18: 623–658.

Habermas, J. 1971. *Knowledge and Human Interests*. Boston: Beacon Press.

Hanly, C. M. T. 1988. Review of *The Foundations of Psychoanalysis* by A. Grünbaum. *Journal of the American Psychoanalytic Association,* 36: 521–528.

Harré, R. 1991. The discursive production of selves. *Theory and Psychology,* 1: 51–63.

Hart, J. E. 1962. *The Red Badge of Courage* as myth and symbol. In S. Bradley et al. (Eds.), *The Red Badge of Courage*. New York: Norton.

Hartmann, H. 1959. Psychoanalysis as a scientific theory. *Essays on Ego Psychology*. New York: International Universities Press, 1964, pp. 318–350.

Hartmann, H., E. Kris, and R. M. Loewenstein. 1946. Comments on the formation of psychic structure. *Psychoanalytic Study of the Child,* 2: 11–38.

Havens, L. 1989. *A Safe Place: Laying the Groundwork for Psychotherapy*. Cambridge: Harvard Univ. Press.

Hobson, J. A. 1988. *The Dreaming Brain*. New York: Basic Books.

Hogben, L. 1943. *Science for the Citizen*. Garden City, N.Y.: Garden City Publishing.

Holt, R. R. 1984. The current status of psychoanalytic theory. Invited address, American Psychological Association, Toronto.

Hook, S. (Ed.). 1959. *Psychoanalysis, Scientific Method, and Philosophy.* New York: New York Univ. Press.

Isay, R. A. 1977. Ambiguity in speech. *Journal of the American Psychoanalytic Association,* 25: 427–452.

Iser, W. 1978. *The Act of Reading.* Baltimore: Johns Hopkins Univ. Press.

Jacobsen, P. B., and R. S. Steele. 1979. From present to past: Freudian archeology. *International Review of Psychoanalysis,* 6: 349–362.

Johan, M. 1985. Reanalysis. *Journal of the American Psychoanalytic Association,* 32: 187–200.

Jones, E. 1953. *The Life and Work of Sigmund Freud,* vol. 1. New York: Basic Books.

Jones, E., and M. Windholz. 1990. The psychoanalytic case study: Toward a method for systematic inquiry. *Journal of the American Psychoanalytic Association,* 38: 371–392.

Kanzer, M., and J. Glenn. (Eds). 1980. *Freud and His Patients.* New York: Aronson.

Kaplan, L. 1978. *Oneness and Separation: From Infant to Individual.* New York: Simon and Schuster.

Kerferd, G. B. 1967. Aristotle. In P. Edwards (Ed.), *The Encyclopedia of Philosophy.* New York: Macmillan.

Kirschner, S. R. 1990. The assenting echo: Anglo-American values in contemporary psychoanalytic developmental psychology. *Social Research,* 57: 821–857.

Klein, G. S. 1976. *Psychoanalytic Theory: An Exploration of Essentials.* New York: International Universities Press.

Klein, M. I., and D. Tribich. 1982. Blame the child. *The Sciences,* 22: 14–20.

Klumpner, G. H., and A. Frank. 1991. On methods of reporting clinical material. *Journal of the American Psychoanalytic Association,* 39: 537–551.

Kohut, H. 1982. Introspection, empathy, and the semicircle of mental health. *International Journal of Psychoanalysis,* 63: 395–407.

Kohut, H. 1984. *How Does Analysis Cure?* Chicago: Univ. of Chicago Press.

Kris, E. 1956. On some vicissitudes of insight. *International Journal of Psychoanalysis,* 37: 445–455.

Kukla, A. 1989. Nonempirical issues in psychology. *American Psychologist,* 44: 785–794.

Lacan, J. 1966. *Ecrits.* Paris: Seuil.

Lear, J. 1990. *Love and Its Place in Nature.* New York: Farrar, Straus & Giroux.

Levy, S. T., and L. B. Inderbitzin. 1990. The analytic surface and the theory of technique. *Journal of the American Psychoanalytic Association,* 38: 371–392.

Lewin, K. 1931. The conflict between Aristotelian and Galilean modes of thought in contemporary psychology. *Journal of General Psychology,* 5: 141–177.

Loewald, H. 1960. On the therapeutic action of psychoanalysis. *International Journal of Psychoanalysis,* 41: 16–33.

Luborsky, L., and D. P. Spence. 1979. Quantitative research on psychoanalytic therapy. In S. L. Garfield and A. E. Bergin (Eds.), *Handbook of Psychotherapy and Behavior Change: An Empirical Analysis.* New York: Wiley.

Mahler, M., F. Pine, and A. Bergman. 1975. *The Psychological Birth of the Human Infant.* New York: Basic Books.

Mahony, P. J. 1987. *Freud as a Writer.* New Haven: Yale Univ. Press.

Masson, J. M. 1984. *The Assault on Truth.* New York: Farrar, Straus & Giroux.

Masson, J. M. 1985. *The Complete Letters of Sigmund Freud to Wilhelm Fliess: 1887–1904.* Cambridge, Mass.: Harvard Univ. Press.

McGrath, W. J. 1986. *Freud's Discovery of Psychoanalysis: The Politics of Hysteria.* Ithaca: Cornell Univ. Press.

McGuire, W. J. 1983. A contextualist theory of knowledge: Its implications for innovation and reform in psychological research. In L. Berkowitz (Ed.), *Advances in Experimental Social Psychology,* vol. 16, pp. 1–47. New York: Academic Press.

McMullin, E. 1967. Empiricism and the scientific revolution. In C. S. Singleton (Ed.), *Art, Science and History in the Renaissance.* Baltimore: Johns Hopkins Univ. Press.

Merton, R. K. 1973. The normative structure of science. In N. W. Storer (Ed.), *The Sociology of Science: Theoretical and Empirical Investigations.* Chicago: Univ. of Chicago Press, pp. 267–278.

Miles, M. B., and A. M. Huberman. 1984. *Qualitative Data Analysis: A Sourcebook of New Methods.* Beverly Hills: Sage Publications.

Murray, H. 1955. Introduction. In A. Burton and R. Harris (Eds.), *Clinical Studies of Personality,* vol. 1. New York: Harper and Row.

Nagel, E. 1959. Methodological issues in psychoanalytic theory. In S. Hook (Ed.), *Psychoanalysis, Scientific Method and Philosophy: A Symposium.* New York: New York Univ. Press, pp. 38–56.

Nehamas, A. 1988. The school of eloquence: Review of Brian Vickers's *In Defense of Rhetoric. Times Literary Supplement,* July 15–21, pp. 771–772.

Ornston, D. 1985. Freud's conception is different from Strachey's. *Journal of the American Psychoanalytic Association,* 33: 379–412.

Packer, M. J., and R. B. Addison. 1989. *Entering the Circle: Hermeneutic Investigation in Psychology.* Albany: State Univ. of New York Press.

Pagels, E. 1979. *The Gnostic Gospels.* New York: Random House.

Paniagua, C. 1985. A methodological approach to surface material. *International Review of Psychoanalysis,* 12: 311–325.

Paniagua, C. 1991. Patient's surface, clinical surface, and workable surface. *Journal of the American Psychoanalytic Association,* 39: 669–685.

Pauley, P. 1988. Review of Anne Harrington's *Medicine, Mind and the Double Brain. Science,* 239: 422.

Pepper, S. C. 1942. *World Hypotheses: A Study in Evidence.* Berkeley: Univ. of California Press.

Poland, W. 1992. From analytic surface to analytic space. *Journal of the American Psychoanalytic Association,* 40: 381–404.

Quine, W. V. O. 1953. Two dogmas of empiricism. In J. Rosenberg and C. Travis (Eds.), *Readings in the Philosophy of Language.* Englewood Cliffs, N.J.: Prentice-Hall, 1971, pp. 63–81.

Quinn, A. 1982. *Figures of Speech: Sixty Ways to Turn a Phrase.* Salt Lake City: Peregrine Smith.

Quinn, S. 1987. *A Mind of Her Own: The Life of Karen Horney.* New York: Summit Books.

Ramzy, I. 1956. From Aristotle to Freud: A few notes on the roots of psychoanalysis. *Bulletin of the Menninger Clinic,* 20: 112–123.

Ramzy, I. 1974. How the mind of the psychoanalyst works: An essay on psychoanalytic inference. *International Journal of Psychoanalysis,* 55: 543–550.

Rangell, L. 1991. Castration. *Journal of the American Psychoanalytic Association,* 39: 3–23.

Reed, G. 1987. Rules of clinical understanding in classical psychoanalysis and self psychology: A comparison. *Journal of the American Psychoanalytic Association,* 35: 421–446.

Reiss, T. J. 1982. *The Discourse of Modernism.* Ithaca: Cornell Univ. Press.

Ricoeur, P. 1970. *Freud and Philosophy.* New Haven: Yale Univ. Press.

Robbins, L. C. 1963. The accuracy of parental recall of aspects of child development and child-rearing practices. *Journal of Abnormal and Social Psychology,* 66: 261–270.

Robinson, R. 1989. *Georgia O'Keeffe.* New York: Harper and Row.

Rorty, R. 1989. *Contingency, Irony and Solidarity.* New York: Cambridge Univ. Press.

Rubovits-Seitz, P. 1988. Kohut's method of interpretation: A critique. *Journal of the American Psychoanalytic Association,* 36: 933–960.

Runyan, W. M. 1984. *Life Histories and Psychobiography.* New York: Oxford Univ. Press.

Rush, B. 1812. *Medical Inquiries and Observations upon the Diseases of the Mind.* Philadelphia: Kinker and Richardson.

Sadoul, J. 1972. *Alchemists and Gold*. Trans. Olga Sieveking. New York: Putnam.

Sampson, E. E. 1981. Cognitive psychology as ideology. *American Psychologist*, 36: 730–743.

Sandler, J., and W. G. Joffe. 1969. On sublimation. In J. Sandler (Ed.), *From Safety to Superego*. New York: Guilford Press, 1987, pp. 235–254.

Schafer, R. 1976. *A New Language for Psychoanalysis*. New Haven: Yale Univ. Press.

Schafer, R. 1985. Wild analysis. *Journal of the American Psychoanalytic Association*, 33: 275–299.

Schimek, J. 1987. Fact and fantasy in the seduction theory: A historical review. *Journal of the American Psychoanalytic Association*, 35: 937–965.

Seelig, B. J. 1993. The analytic surface. *Journal of the American Psychoanalytic Association*, 41: 179–190.

Simon, B. 1991. Is the Oedipus complex still the cornerstone of psychoanalysis? Three obstacles to answering the question. *Journal of the American Psychoanalytic Association*, 39: 641–668.

Simon, B. 1992. "Incest—see under Oedipus Complex": The history of an error in psychoanalysis. *Journal of the American Psychoanalytic Association*, 40: 955–988.

Skinner, B. F. 1987. Whatever happened to psychology as a science of behavior? *American Psychologist*, 42: 780–786.

Smith, J. 1657. *The Mysterie of Rhetorique Unvail'd*. London: Menston (facsimile edition).

Southern, R. W. 1953. *The Making of the Middle Ages*. New Haven: Yale Univ. Press.

Spence, D. P. 1973. Analogue and digital descriptions of behavior. *American Psychologist*, 28: 479–488.

Spence, D. P. 1981. Toward a theory of dream interpretation. *Psychoanalysis and Contemporary Thought*, 4: 383–405.

Spence, D. P. 1982. *Narrative Truth and Historical Truth*. New York: W. W. Norton.

Spence, D. P. 1987. *The Freudian Metaphor*. New York: W. W. Norton.

Spence, D. P. 1992. Interpretation: A critical perspective. In J. W. Barron, M. N. Eagle, and D. L. Wolitzky (Eds.), *Interface of Psychoanalysis and Psychology*. Washington, D.C.: American Psychological Association.

Spence, D. P. and B. Holland. 1962. The restricting effects of awareness: A paradox and an explanation. *Journal of Abnormal and Social Psychology*, 64: 163–174.

Spence, D. P., H. S. Scarborough, and E. H. Ginsberg. 1978. Lexical correlates of cervical cancer. *Social Science and Medicine*, 12: 141–145.

Spence, D. P., L. C. Mayes, and H. Dahl. (in press). Monitoring the analytic surface. *Journal of the American Psychoanalytic Association.*

Spencer, J. H., Jr., and L. Balter. 1990. Psychoanalytic observation. *Journal of the American Psychoanalytic Association,* 38: 393–421.

Spock, B. 1945. *Baby and Child Care.* New York: Pocket Books.

Stein, M. 1988. Writing about psychoanalysis: I. Analysts who write and those who do not. *Journal of the American Psychoanalytic Association,* 36: 105–124.

Stoller, R. J. 1988. Patients' responses to their own case reports. *Journal of the American Psychoanalytic Association,* 36: 371–391.

Stolorow, R. D. and G. E. Atwood. 1979. *Faces in the Cloud.* New York: Jason Aronson.

Strachey, J. 1934. The nature of the therapeutic action of psychoanalysis. *International Journal of Psychoanalysis,* 15: 127–159.

Sulloway, F. 1979. *Freud, Biologist of the Mind.* New York: Basic Books.

Sulloway, F. 1991. Reassessing Freud's case histories: The social construction of psychoanalysis. *Isis,* 82: 245–275.

Templkin, O. 1952. The elusiveness of Paracelsus. *Bulletin of the History of Medicine,* 26: 201–217.

Toews, J. E. 1991. Historicizing psychoanalysis: Freud in our time and for our time. *Journal of Modern History,* 63: 504–545.

Tracy, D. 1981. *The Analogical Imagination.* New York: Crossroad.

Vickers, B. (Ed.) 1984. *Occult and Scientific Mentalities in the Renaissance.* Cambridge: Cambridge Univ. Press.

Vickers, B. 1988. *In Defence of Rhetoric.* Oxford: Oxford Univ. Press.

Viderman, S. 1979. Interpretation in the analytic space. *International Review of Psychoanalysis,* 1: 467–480.

Walker, D. P. 1958. *Spiritual and Demonic Magic from Ficino to Campanella.* London.

Wallerstein, R. S. 1988. One psychoanalysis or many? *International Journal of Psychoanalysis,* 69: 5–21.

Waugaman, R. M. 1990. On patients' disclosure of parents' and siblings' names during treatment. *Journal of the American Psychoanalytic Association,* 38: 167–194.

Wear, A., R. K. French, and I. M. Lonie (Eds.). 1985. *The Medical Renaissance of the Sixteenth Century.* Cambridge: Cambridge Univ. Press.

Weiss, T. (unpublished). At the mercy of the play: Poetry and its discontents.

Westfall, R. S. 1984. Newton and alchemy. In B. Vickers (Ed.), *Occult and Scientific Mentalities in the Renaissance.* Cambridge: Cambridge Univ. Press.

White, H. 1978. *Tropics of Discourse.* Baltimore: Johns Hopkins Univ. Press.
Williams, M. 1987. Reconstruction of an early seduction and its aftereffects. *Journal of the American Psychoanalytic Association,* 35: 145–163.
Wurmser, L. 1977. A defense of the use of metaphor in analytic theory formation. *Psychoanalytic Quarterly,* 46: 466–498.

Index

Action, 57
Adler, Alfred, 4, 93, 150–151, 169
Aemulatio, 58, 61–62, 65–66
Aeneid, 104
Affection, 65
Alchemy, 3, 41, 42, 105–106, 113, 125–127, 129, 130, 141
Allusion, 35, 62, 98, 99, 100, 108
Ambassadors, The (James), 131
American Psychoanalytic Association, 90
Analogue reasoning, 52
Analogy, 31, 57–63, 78–79, 127, 180
Analysand. *See* Patient
Analytic hour, 4, 61, 68, 137, 153, 156, 159, 188, 189–190, 203. *See also* "Good hour"
Analytic process: features of, 24–25; as history taking, 71, 116–117; anthropomorphism in, 80–82; artifacts in, 92; suggestion in, 92–93, 113, 122, 130, 133–134, 169, 179; inference in, 118–119, 133–134; restrictions on, 123, 128–129, 147–148; failures of, 124, 129; notes, 149–150, 154, 186, 191–192; timing in, 153, 159, 186–194; patterns in, 159–162, 186–194, 197, 198–199; as archeology, 167–169, 178; phases in, 190, 194
Analytic sequence, 159–161
Analytic space, 25, 137, 184, 186–189, 190–194, 199

Analytic surface, 25, 89, 183–194, 196, 197, 199, 200–204
Analyzing instrument, 119, 135, 194
Anecdote, 2–4, 15, 119, 121, 123, 145–148, 150, 154, 157–158, 186, 191–192, 195–197
Anthropomorphism, 80–82
Antipathy, 64, 65
Archeology, 32, 95, 167–169, 178
Argument by authority: power of, 1–4, 12, 25, 30–32, 34–35, 40–41, 91–94, 97, 99, 108–111, 114–116, 146, 155, 194; results of, 23–25, 103–105, 107, 119–120, 122–124, 132; secrecy and, 125–128, 129–130, 139–141
Aristotelian science: single specimens in, 1–3, 39–41, 48–54, 56, 67–68, 71–74, 88–91, 97, 110–116, 130, 134, 136–141, 147, 150, 152, 158, 179, 195–196; expert observers in, 40–41, 46, 51, 55, 60–61, 74, 90, 91, 94, 110–117, 122–123, 126, 134, 140–141; theory and, 42–54, 114, 115; methods of, 57–69, 72–74, 77, 94, 106, 109–110, 113–114; metaphor and, 89–90
Aristotle, 1–2, 23, 37, 39, 40, 47, 50, 57, 60, 62
Associations: phonetic, 35–36; semantic, 35–36; context of, 36–38, 70; vs. causation, 38, 46; interpretation of, 45, 46, 61, 69–72; sequence of, 61; free, 62, 92, 106, 113; importance of, 65,

Associations (*continued*)
66, 69, 168; coherence and 69–72;
composite objects in, 71; dreams and
98–99; analysand and, 186
Astington, J. W., 196
Astrology, 56–57, 126
Atwood, G. E., 170–171

Baby and Child Care (Spock), 14
Background repetition, 187
Bacon, Sir Francis, 29, 41, 51, 105, 110,
113, 182
Baconian Revolution, 1–2, 29, 41, 51,
54, 105–106, 110, 128–129, 158
Balter, Leon, 194
Bauhim, Casper, 51
Bernstein, R. J., 87
Biography, 170–173
Boesky, Dale, 183–184
Bonaparte, Maria, 102, 106
Botanical medicine, 126
Botanical Monograph dream, 35–36, 37
Bowie, Malcolm, 167, 168, 169
Boyd, Richard, 84
Boyle, Robert, 29, 45, 127
Brentano, Franz, 47, 54
Brain hemispheres, 166–167
Brenner, Charles, 2, 128
Breuer, Josef, 14
"Broken heart," 165, 166
Broyard, Anatole, 63
Brücke, Ernst, 29
Burton, Richard, 38

Campbell, D. T., 125, 126, 139
Cartesian anxiety, 87
Case histories: anecdotal, 2–3, 15, 119,
121, 123, 145–148, 150, 154,
157–158, 186, 191–192, 196–197;
seduction theory and, 3–4, 14–16, 24,
124, 131–140; ambiguity in, 3, 43,
94, 118–122, 129–135, 141,
146–148; verbatim, 30, 90, 118–121,
129–130, 133, 140, 147, 191; Anna
O., 40; Dora, 43, 49, 79, 97, 114,
118, 145; influence of, 46–47, 80,
91–94, 118–124, 145–146, 163;
guidelines for, 90, 119, 191–194;

Wolf Man, 92, 93, 118, 157, 169;
necessary truths in, 120, 134; contingent truths in, 120, 135, 136,
191–192; modern, 121; singular
explanation in, 121–122, 138; as literature, 135, 169, 197–198; disagreement over, 122–123, 129; facts in,
122–123, 129, 131, 132–134,
136–138, 147, 158; expert opinion in,
122–123, 140–141; unsuccessful analyses in, 124, 129; self-serving, 124,
145–148, 157–158; protection by disguise in, 129, 147–148, 195; Freudian
voice in, 131–132, 136, 139–140,
145, 195; analyst thoughts in, 131,
133–140; quality of, 135, 140–141,
145–146, 158–159, 195–197; function of, 145–146, 163; incomplete,
146–154, 158–159, 163, 185, 195;
public reporting on, 152–159; representative, 157–159; Rat Man, 157,
169; as training, 163; Mrs. C., 186,
189–194, 197, 198, 201
Castration anxiety, 198
Cavell, Marcia, 69, 70
Cerebral palsy, 29–30
Chiasmus, 85
Child abuse. *See* Seduction theory;
Sexual abuse
Civilization and Its Discontents (Freud),
167
Clark, Ronald, 21, 33
Class membership, 50, 53, 57, 60
Clinical archive, 11, 30, 90–91, 168,
195, 197. *See also* Public data base
Clinical surface, 185, 193, 199
Clinician's Fallacy, 156
Coherence theory, 69, 70–74, 120, 154
Columbus, Christopher, 176
Communality, 162–163
Competence, 115–116, 119, 122–123
Computer analysis, 150, 154, 186,
189–193
Conceptualism. *See* Aristotelian science
Confidentiality, 12, 24, 105, 123,
128–129, 147–148, 162, 195
Confirmation-biased research, 161–162
Connaître, 200

Contemporary root metaphors, 166, 170, 173–180
Contiguity, 58, 61, 156, 194
Contingent features, 53–54, 60, 67–69, 72–74, 90, 94, 120–121, 135, 136, 159, 162, 191–192
Convenientia, 58, 61
Cooper, S. H., 187
Copernican system, 9, 202, 203
Core specimens. *See* Specimen cases
Correlation analysis, 187–194, 198, 201, 202
Correspondence theory, 69, 70–74, 120, 154
CORtrans, 188–189
Cortical control, 166–167
Countertransference, 122, 140, 185, 191, 197
Count Thun dream, 37
Crews, Frederick, 101–102, 112, 115
Crollius, 58
Cuddon, J. A., 77
Cultural context, 166–170, 177, 178–180

Darwin, Charles, 21, 28, 38
Davidson, Donald, 70
Debus, A. G., 50–51
Deconstructionist critique, 92–93, 178–179
Defense mechanisms, 183, 191, 192
Depth, 194, 197
Derivatives, 61–62, 192–193, 197, 199
Descartes, René, 42, 87
Dewey, John, 175
Dialectical tradition, 3, 122
Dialogue, 90, 118, 121, 140, 191–192
Digital reasoning, 52
Dinnage, Rosemary, 195
Doctrine of Signatures: transformations and, 54–60, 62, 64; categories and, 58, 60–68; arbitrary nature of, 60–61, 63–69
Dream(s): wish fulfillment in, 2, 11, 20–21, 35, 45, 79, 98–100, 103, 110, 129; seduction theory and, 18, 19, 133–136; Mathilde, 19; literature of, 27–28, 34–36, 98, 118; specimen, 27, 30, 34, 36–38, 45, 46, 52–54, 56, 72, 74, 104, 108, 114, 115; accessibility of, 30, 36–38; Botanical Monograph, 35–36, 37; Count Thun, 37; Irma, 37, 49, 53, 56, 74, 79, 97, 114; examination, 53, 54; latent, 55, 98; manifest, 55, 98–99; coherence analysis and 72; as past events, 98–99, 103, 106–107, 131–136, 167–169; repetitive, 133, 134
Dream formation: laws of, 2, 131–132, 136; analysis of, 27–28, 34–38, 45, 46, 61, 98–100, 131–133; signature analysis and, 55, 56; similitudes and, 61
"Dreckology reports," 16
Drive mechanisms, 191
Dynamic surface, 183

Eckstein, Emma, 13
Egalitarianism, 125, 139
Ego and the Id, The (Freud), 167
Eissler, Kurt, 2, 100–101, 114, 116
Elitism, 40–41, 46, 51, 55, 60–61, 74, 90, 91, 94, 110–123, 126, 128, 134, 140–141, 163. *See also* Aristotelian science
Ellenberger, Henri, 29–30, 101
Emde, R. N., 22
Emotions, 165, 166, 170
Empathy, 63, 82, 86–87, 197
Empirical psychology, 39, 87, 109–110, 113–114, 179
Empiricism. *See* Galilean science
Enactment, 197
Enargia, 33–34, 85, 86, 109, 120, 130, 138, 139
Epistemic access, 84, 86, 91, 177. *See also* Vanishing referent
Erikkson, Ruben, 51
Essences, 57–61, 64
Ethnography, 31–32
Evidential surface, 197–199, 201–202
Evidential voice: metaphor vs., 2, 35–36, 62, 77–79, 81–88, 91, 93–94, 127, 129, 155, 165–170; power of, 87–89, 95–96, 99–100, 104,

Evidential voice (*continued*)
    155–162, 180–182; description and,
    89–91, 94–99, 197–199, 201
Examination dream, 53, 54
Examples. *See* Specimen cases
Experimentation, 52, 72–74, 77,
    124–126

Fantasy: sexual, 3–4, 10–11, 17, 19–21;
    role of, 3–4, 12–13, 43, 71; con-
    scious, 17; importance of, 17, 19,
    20–21, 43, 68, 71; unconscious, 17,
    21, 43
Felman, Shoshana, 10
Feminine development, 22, 176–177
Ferenczi, Sándor, 151
Fiction: fact vs., 164–166, 169–170,
    178–179, 181; American, 174–178;
    root metaphors in, 174–178
Fiedler, Leslie, 175–176
First names, 149–150, 154–161
Firth, Raymond, 31–32
Fish, Stanley, 92–93, 165–166, 180
Fisher, Seymour, 22
Flexner, Abraham, 25–26, 148–149
Fliess, Wilhelm, 43–44, 106
Fliess correspondence: on oedipal
    theory, 11, 14, 17; on seduction
    theory, 15–16, 18–20, 21, 42; on *Die
    Traumdeutung*, 27, 33, 35, 38, 97,
    98; on self-analysis, 100–102, 104,
    108; on Bellevue, 104
'Folk psychology,' 204
Foreground repetition, 187
Foucault, Michel, 54, 55–56, 57–59
Foundations of Psychoanalysis, The
    (Grünbaum), 112–115
"Fragments of an Analysis of a Case of
    Hysteria" (Freud), 167–168
Frank, Alvin, 90
Free associations, 62, 92, 106, 113
Free-floating attention, 194
Freud, Anna, 17, 102, 106
Freud, Jakob, 18–20
Freud, Julius, 171
Freud, Mathilde, 19
Freud, Sigmund: seduction theory and,
    1, 3–4, 14–24, 42, 43, 44, 52–53, 77,
    106, 135–136, 158, 169; case histo-
    ries of, 1–3, 14–16, 24, 30, 40, 43,
    46, 79–80, 91–93, 97, 114, 118,
    120–124, 130, 135, 145–148, 155,
    157, 163, 169; scientific method and,
    1–3, 23–25, 29–30, 37–40, 42–48,
    52–54, 77–83, 89, 103–115, 128,
    145, 163, 173, 179; influence of,
    1–4, 17, 23–25, 30–31, 46–48,
    79–80, 83, 88, 91–96, 99–107,
    111–117, 124, 132, 139–140,
    145–148, 155–158, 203; self-analysis
    of, 2, 16, 19–20, 28, 30, 44, 49,
    97–105, 106–117, 167, 171–173,
    179–180; biographers of, 2, 19–21,
    39, 97, 100–117, 150–151, 171–173,
    180–181; on dreaming, 2, 27–28,
    35–38, 45, 54, 72, 79, 98–100,
    104–105, 106, 109, 131–132; on
    reconstruction, 2, 95, 98–102,
    131–132, 167–169; oedipal theory
    and, 10–11, 17–24, 25, 106, 107,
    171–172, 178, 203; on remembering,
    11, 14, 95, 98–101, 131–132,
    167–168; father and, 18–19; dreams
    of, 18, 19, 20–21, 35–36, 98–100,
    104, 105, 108; personal history of,
    18–22, 23, 33, 43, 171–173, 178,
    180; mother and, 19–20, 99, 171; as
    explorer/hero, 21, 27–39, 97–98,
    100–105, 108, 114–117, 180–182,
    195; on male development, 22; uni-
    versal phenomenon and, 23, 40, 46,
    98–99, 171–173; narrative skill of,
    30–36, 78–80, 85–86, 88, 91–93,
    95–97, 117, 120–121, 135, 169, 180,
    194–195, 196; as archeologist, 32,
    95, 167–169, 178; signature analysis
    and, 54–55, 56; free associations and,
    62, 92, 106, 113; coherence analysis
    and, 72; autobiography of, 102; note-
    books of, 108; on Dora case, 118; on
    patient privacy, 123, 147–148; on
    Adler, 150–151, 169; on Jung, 151,
    169; on timing, 153; training analysis
    and, 163; on mental forces, 165;
    industrial revolution and, 170; on
    analytic surface, 184, 186

Freudian Metaphor, The (Spence), 90–91
Freudian politics, 150, 202
Freudian slips, 55, 180
Future of an Illusion, The (Freud), 167

Gadamer, Hans-Georg, 94
Galilean science: public debate in, 2, 43, 93, 103–104, 122–125, 128–130, 139–140, 147, 162; methods of, 39, 41–53, 67–69, 109–110, 113–114, 124–125, 199; theory in, 42–54, 87–90, 120; evidence in, 111–116, 135, 139–141, 146–147, 158; sample size in, 111, 149, 179; metaphor in, 127; clinical science vs., 145–147, 196, 199; norms of, 162–163
Galileo, 21, 41, 42, 48, 113
Gardner, Howard, 170
Gay, Peter, 112, 150–151, 180, 181; on seduction theory, 21; on scientific method, 39; on self-analysis, 49, 101, 104–105, 108–111, 114–117, 171, 173; on oedipal theory, 171–172
Geertz, Clifford, 31–32, 89, 120
Gender Identity, 22
Genotype, 51–52, 54, 60
Gergen, Kenneth J., 86, 164–165
Gergen, Mary, 164–165
Glenn, Jules, 121
Gnosis, 200–202
Goldberger, Miriam, 183
"Good Bad Boy," 175–176
"Good hour," 12–13, 14, 74
Gray, Paul, 184
Greenberg, R. P., 22
Greenwald, A. G., 159–160, 161–162, 177
Grief, 165, 166
Grillparzer, Franz, 11
Grossman, W. I., 81–82, 84
Grünbaum, Adolf, 39, 112–115, 128, 157, 180

Habermas, Jürgen, 3, 126, 140, 194
Hanly, C. M. T., 113
Hannibal, 32–33
Harré, Rom, 187

Harris, P. L., 196
Hartmann, Heinz, 80–81, 82, 84, 88, 89
Harvey, William, 113
Hawking, Stephen, 164
Heraclitus, 103
Hermeneutics, 77, 178–179, 195, 196
Heroic legends, 97, 101–105, 114–117, 174–177, 180–181
Hobson, J. A., 112
Hogben, Lancelot, 9
Holt, R. R., 128
Home base, 174, 175, 176
Hook, Sidney, 115
Huberman, A. M., 70
Human nature, 101, 103, 111, 121, 170–171
Hume, David, 54
Hyperbole, 155
Hypothesis-testing method, 159–160
Hysteria, 14–19, 42, 102

Incest, 11, 20–21, 24, 146, 155. *See also* Oedipal theory
Inderbitzin, L. B., 184, 194
Infant development, 173–177, 178
Infantile wishes, 2, 11, 20–21, 35, 45, 79, 98–100, 103, 110, 129
Interpretation: credibility of, 11, 34–38, 67–68, 72–74, 79, 91–95, 97–99, 103–104, 114, 118–119, 134, 147–148, 154; mutative, 25; inexact, 25, 148; unlimited, 48–49, 56; signs and, 54–60; similitudes and, 61–68, 138; as cure, 66, 67, 68, 79, 200; generalization vs., 74, 94–95, 103, 111, 134; sectarian, 148–149, 155–156; timing of, 153, 186–194, 198, 201, 203
Interpretation of Dreams, The (Freud). *See Traumdeutung, Die*
Intervention frequency, 153, 186–194, 198, 201, 203
Introductory Lectures (Freud), 93
Intuition, 1, 24, 39–40, 46, 52, 57–58, 63, 74, 77, 86
Irma dream, 37, 49, 53, 56, 74, 79, 97, 114

Jacobsen, P. B., 107
Johan, Morton, 66
Jones, Enrico, 189
Jones, Ernest, 2, 19, 39, 150–151; on oedipal theory, 20–21; on self-analysis, 100–103, 108–109, 110, 114, 116, 117
Jung, Carl, 1, 4, 40, 77, 93, 150, 151, 169, 171

Kanzer, Mark, 121
Kennen, 200
Klein, M. I., 118
Kleinian theory, 198
Klumpner, G. H., 90
Knowledge: theory vs., 24–26; metaphor vs., 84–89, 93, 127, 129, 166, 170, 201, 203–204; reflective, 167, 200
Krafft-Ebing, Richard von, 15
Kris, Ernst, 12–13, 74, 81, 102, 106
Kukla, Andre, 54, 67

Language: pictorial, 30–36, 72–74, 78–80, 85–93, 120, 158–159, 180; faults, 55; analysis of, 62, 153, 186–194; action, 82; things vs., 127–128, 129, 146; scientific, 140, 186, 194, 196–197, 201–204; constraints on, 166; cultural context of, 169–170, 178–179; imprecise, 183–186, 202–203; patterns, 186–194, 197; *spatial location* and, 187, 188; *temporal moment* and, 187, 188; intimacy and, 189; private, 195, 200. *See also* Narrative; Rhetoric
Latent content, 55–56, 57, 58, 65, 98, 137, 153
Latent surface, 184
Latent trigger, 191
Lawfulness, 50, 53, 159, 197, 203
Levy, S. T., 184
Lewin, Kurt, 40, 50, 51, 60
Literature, 62, 121, 135, 164, 169, 174–177, 178, 197–198
Loewenstein, R. M., 81
Logic, 1, 3, 36, 43, 77, 153, 155–156, 158–162
Luborsky, Lester, 200

Macrocosm, 56–57, 58, 59
Mahler, Margaret, 173–177, 178
Mahony, Patrick J., 27, 34, 39–40, 77, 85, 96, 180
Manifest content, 55–56, 57, 58, 60, 98–99, 153
Manifest surface, 184
Manifest trigger, 191
Marker words, 187–194, 197, 198
Masculine development, 22, 174–177
'Masculine protest,' 150
Masson, Jeffrey, 15, 27, 33, 35, 97, 98, 102, 104; on seduction theory, 4, 16–17, 19; on oedipal theory, 11, 14, 19–20; Freud Archives and, 16
Master-apprentice tradition, 46–47, 200
McGrath, W. J., 33
McGuire, W. J., 159, 161
McMullin, Ernan, 40–41, 42, 45–46, 50, 51, 110, 111
McPhee, John, 164
Meaning, 55–60
Medical education, 25–26, 148–149
Medicine, 25–26, 50, 57, 59–60, 148–149
Memories: early childhood, 2, 3–4, 15–18, 95, 98–101, 104, 107, 131–138; recovery of, 2, 12, 95, 98–101, 104, 131–138, 167–169; theory and, 11–14, 15, 17–18; affective charge and, 12, 13; critical, 25; interpretation and, 61; power of, 167; preservation of, 167–169
Mental modules theory, 170
Mental processes: inaccessibility of, 28, 62, 84, 86–87, 93, 128, 165–166, 170, 172–173, 179; primary, 35–37, 45, 55, 87, 194; secondary, 45, 87; as social myth, 86–87, 170, 174–180; dissection and, 165, 166; preservation in, 168–169
Mental process theories: mechanical, 82; metaphor and, 83, 85–87, 166, 173–180; archeology and, 95, 167–169, 178; human anatomy and, 165, 166, 170; cultural influences on, 166–170, 177, 178–180; personal history and, 166, 170–173, 177, 179,

180; artificial intelligence and, 170; industrial revolution and, 170; infancy and, 173–177, 178; as fiction, 178–179

Merton, R. K., 162

Metalepsis, 107–108, 129, 130, 138, 139, 155

Metaphoric surface, 183

Metaphors: of Freud, 2, 27–29, 31, 78–81, 83, 85, 86, 88, 95–96, 168–169, 170, 194–195; evidence and, 2, 35–36, 62, 78–79, 81–88, 127, 129, 155, 165–170; appeal of, 2, 85–87, 93–96, 165–166, 169–170, 180, 185–186, 194, 196; replacement of, 79, 80–89, 91, 95, 166, 194; science and, 82–83, 87–89, 91, 127, 130, 194–195, 201, 203–204; referent vs., 83–87, 93, 127, 129, 146, 165–166, 194–195; dead, 83, 88; choice of, 83, 170; as fact, 84, 89, 93, 127, 129, 166, 170, 201, 203–204; telescope, 86; root, 166, 170, 173–178; young male hero, 174–177, 178; New World discoverer, 174–177

Metapsychology, 25, 82–83, 170–171

Metatheory, 82–83

Metonomy, 78, 107, 130

Microcosm, 57, 58, 59

Middle Ages, 50–51, 54–60, 73–74, 105–106, 138. *See also* Aristotelian science; Occult

Miles, M. B., 70

Mill, John Stuart, 43, 113

"Mover of the mental apparatus," 165

Mrs. C. case, 186, 189–194, 197, 198, 201

Murray, Henry, 121

'Mutual monitoring,' 126

Mysticism, 40, 151, 167

Myth, 5, 9–14, 17, 23–26, 86–87, 97–104, 108, 115–117, 174–182, 196

Nagel, Ernest, 81, 86, 115

Naming behavior. *See* First names

Narrative: persuasiveness of, 13, 30–36, 73–74, 79, 85, 91–96, 118–121, 135, 158–159, 169, 172, 178–179; coher-

ence of, 13, 72–74, 80, 95–96; selectivity in, 119–124, 146–154, 158–159; personal history and, 172–173

'Narrative fit,' 79, 131

Natural history, 27–32, 35–39

Necessary features, 53–54, 66, 67–69, 91, 120, 134, 159, 161, 162

Nehamas, Alexander, /8, 11/

Neurosis, *neurotica*. *See* Hysteria

Newton, Sir Isaac, 41–42, 45–46, 48, 49

Newtonian revolution, 150

New World discoverer myth, 174–177

Normal science. *See* Galilean science

"Normative Structure of Science, The" (Merton), 162

Occult: sciences, 3, 105–106, 108, 113, 125–130, 141; theory of gravity and, 11, influence of, 12, 151, 195; signature analysis and, 56–57; classification, 91. *See also* Alchemy

Oedipal theory: acceptance of, 4, 21–23, 25; universality and, 10–11, 19–24, 25, 171–172, 173, 178, 198; seduction theory and, 14, 17–24; fantasy and, 17, 20–21; clinical data and, 22–23, 149–150, 154, 155, 156, 158, 161, 202–203; family environment and, 22, 171–172, 173, 178; self-analysis and, 106, 107, 171–172, 173; first names and, 149–150, 154, 155, 156, 158, 161

Oedipus myth, 10–11, 17, 33, 172

Olson, D. R., 196

Omnipotent fusion, 173–174

On the History of the Psychoanalytic Movement (Freud), 98

Openings, 192–193, 197, 199

Pagels, Elaine, 200

Paniagua, Cecilio, 184–186, 193, 194, 196, 199

Paracelsian principles, 126–127

Paracelsus, 55, 60

Parallel processing, 170

Paraphrase, 90, 121, 140

Participatory democracy, 2, 29, 51, 105–107, 113, 122–125, 128–130, 139

Passion, 57

Patient: self-analysis, 12, 13; privacy, 12, 24, 105, 123, 128–129, 147–148, 162, 195; as statistic, 69; testimony, 90–91, 137, 140; viewpoint, 90–91, 161; analyst relationship, 113, 137–138, 147–148, 161, 183–194, 198, 200–201, 204; initial diagnosis of, 119; self-knowledge, 183–184; associations, 186; repetition, 187; pronoun use, 187–194

Pattern-finding method, 159–162

Pattern matches. *See* Similitudes

Pauley, P., 166–167

Pearlstein, Philip, 63

Pensée pensante, 96

Phallocentrism, 178

Phenomenal surface, 183

Phenotype, 40, 51–52, 54, 60

Philosopher's Stone, 105

Philosophy of science, 161

Place, 57, 65

Plato, 78, 93–94

Poetry, 86, 195, 196

Poland, Warren, 183, 184

Positivism, 39, 44, 96, 122, 130, 148–152, 157–162

Posture, 57

Practicing subphase, 174

Primary-process thinking, 35–37, 45, 55, 87, 194, Privileged competence, 119, 122–123

Privileged withholding, 122–123, 147–148, 185, 195

Probability, 52

Processive style, 96

Projection, 198

Projective fallacy, 72

Pronoun markers, 187–194, 197, 198, 201, 202

Prototype, 50

Proximity, 58, 61

Psychic reality, 17, 42, 71, 169

Psychic structure, 25, 201

Psychoanalysis: purpose of, 62, 183; described, 88–89; integrity of, 92–93, 111–112, 115–117; autonomy of, 92, 163; secret sources in, 105–108, 110, 114, 117, 130, 141; as faith, 112, 117, 130, 141, 179–182, 195, 203; as archeology, 167–169, 178; research and, 195–196, 200

Psychoanalysts: as empiricists, 2, 67–69, 89, 128–130, 135, 179–180; clinical data and, 11–13, 14, 23–25, 49, 67–74, 89–91, 95, 118–123, 131–136, 152–163, 186–194; personal history of, 12, 13, 18–21, 69, 111, 119, 122, 130, 136, 166, 170–173, 177, 178, 196, 198–199, 200, 204; self-protection and, 12, 123, 147–148; as conceptualists, 46, 49, 55, 57, 67–69, 73–74, 89–90, 106, 111, 114–117, 128–130, 136–137; transformations and, 55, 57, 62; similitudes and, 61–68, 156; plausibility and, 70; consciousness of, 70, 71–73, 186, 191–192, 197, 200–201, 204; inexperienced, 71; suggestion and, 92–93, 113, 122, 130, 133–134; average, 114; competence of, 115–116, 119, 122–123; incomplete reporting and, 146–154, 158–159, 163, 185; numbers of, 149, 154; role confusion and, 152–159; as archeologists, 167–169, 178; analytic surface and, 183–194; analytic space and, 184, 186–194; classical, 189–190, 198

Psychoanalytic argument, 2, 77

Psychoanalytic glossaries, 183, 197, 204

Psychoanalytic literature: language of, 30–36, 72–74, 77–81, 88, 90–94, 96, 140, 194–195, 197–198, 201–204; core specimens in, 48, 72–74, 90–94, 129–130, 145, 155–158; similitudes in, 63–66, 156; contingent features in, 67, 90, 94, 120, 135, 159; coherence analysis and, 72–74, 154; patient testimony in, 90–91, 137, 140; reader demands of, 94–95, 162, 163; Freudian critiques in, 112–117, 151, 179–182; evolution of, 120–124, 130,

145–146, 157–158, 181–182,
191–204; necessary features in, 120,
134, 159, 161; singular explanation
in, 121–122, 123, 138; self-serving,
124, 145–148, 157–158; incomplete
reporting in, 146–152, 158–159, 163,
185, 195; public reporting in,
152–159; quality of, 158–159, 162,
195; private reporting in, 161,
200–201. *See also* Case histories
Psychoanalytic theory: criticisms of, 4,
23–25, 91, 95–96, 103–104, 106,
111–117, 123–124, 145–148, 151,
179–182; as myth, 5, 10–13, 23–25,
86–87, 97–104, 108, 115–117,
174–182, 196; personal history and,
18–23, 69, 111, 166, 170–181, 196,
198–199; as metaphor, 83–89, 146;
validity of, 113–114, 116, 158,
179–180; proof and, 128, 133–134,
146, 148, 155–159; sectarian,
148–152, 155–158, 162
Psychoanalytic training, 46–47, 92, 163,
183, 200
Psychobiography, 170–173
Psychological birth, 173–174, 175
Psychological relativism, 198
Psychotherapy Process Q-sort, 189
Ptolemaic system, 9, 10, 202, 203
Public data base: importance of, 1–2,
105–107, 122–130; accessibility to, 3,
11, 24, 30, 74, 91, 110, 112, 119,
139–140, 146–147, 162; lack of, 12,
15, 43, 134, 195

Quality, 57, 64, 65, 66
Quantity, 57
Quine, W. V. O., 201
Quintilian, 33–34

Ramzy, Ishak, 39, 47, 152–153
Rangell, Leo, 198
Rank, Otto, 171
Rapprochement subphase, 174
Rationality, 167, 200
Reconstruction, 2, 95, 98–102, 104,
131–133, 134, 136–138, 167–169
"Reconstruction of an Early Seduction

and Its Aftereffects" (Williams),
131–140, 157, 158, 162
Reed, Gail, 64, 65
Referent. *See* Metaphors; Vanishing referent
Reich, Wilhelm, 171
Reiss, T. J., 49
Relation, 57
Religion, 40, 151
Remembering process, 11, 13–14, 15,
95, 98–101, 103, 106–107, 131–136,
167–169
Renaissance, 3, 24, 39, 40, 48, 53, 54,
56, 67, 106, 110, 114, 122, 125. *See
also* Galilean science
Repetition, 50, 126, 133, 134, 187
Replication: importance of, 1, 3, 36–38,
41, 48, 52, 54, 56, 67–73, 128–129,
195, 202; repetition vs. 50, 126; signature analysis and, 60–61, 63–64,
67–69; context and, 70–73, 161–162;
need for, 104, 110–115, 124–125,
130, 179–181
Repression, 11, 84, 100, 150
Resemblance. *See* Similitudes
Resistance, 106
Rhetoric: figurative language in, 33–36,
80, 85–87, 120–121, 130; general
laws and, 37–38, 80–89, 91, 94, 96,
152, 157–161, 179–182, 184, 186;
similitudes and, 62, 138; experimentation vs., 72–74, 77, 127, 129–130;
defined, 77–78; reason vs., 77, 78, 85,
117; as phase, 77, 79, 81–83, 88–89,
95; figures of speech in, 78–79,
85–86, 88, 95–96, 103, 107–108,
127, 130, 138, 139, 186, 201; decline
of, 78, 81–89, 91, 93–96; analytic
technique and, 79, 133–134,
137–141; empty, 91–96, 127–128;
causal explanations vs., 94–97,
127–129, 134–139, 158–161,
178–179, 194, 196; legends and, 97,
101–105, 114–117; secrecy and,
105–110, 117, 125–130; history vs.,
116–117; reductive, 126–131,
134–135; descriptive, 127, 130; personal history and, 172–173

Rhetorical figures. *See* Argument by
   authority; *Chiasmus; Enargia; Hyper-*
   bole; Metalepsis; Metaphors; *Syl-*
   lepsis; Tropes
Ricoeur, Paul, 94, 135
Robbins, Lillian, 13–14, 15
Royal Society, 24, 29, 51, 113
Rush, Benjamin, 165, 166

Sadoul, J., 105–106
Sample size: importance of, 29, 39,
   110–114, 153–159, 179; research
   and, 41, 48, 50–54; description of,
   149–150
Sampson, Edward, 87, 170
Savoir, 200
Sceptical Chymist (Boyle), 29
Schafer, Roy, 71, 79, 82, 165
Schimek, Jean, 15, 17
Scientific method: induction and, 1–3,
   24, 29, 39–45, 52–54, 68–69, 77,
   79–81, 87–88, 113, 124–125, 199;
   general laws and, 37–38, 41, 44–51,
   56, 67–74, 79, 80–83, 87–88, 91,
   114; quantification and, 41, 52, 82,
   110–111, 114, 120, 149–150,
   153–159, 179; clinical acumen and,
   115–116; bias and, 148–149, 154,
   161–162, 177–178, 196; record-
   keeping in, 149–150, 154; reality and,
   164–166. *See also* Galilean science
Scientific revolution, 1–2, 29, 41, 42,
   51, 54, 105–106, 110, 128–129, 150,
   158
Secondary-process thinking, 45, 87
Secrecy. *See* Argument by authority;
   Occult
Sectarianism, 148–152, 155–157, 162
Seduction theory: revision of, 1, 3–4,
   14–24, 42, 43, 52, 106; fantasy and,
   3–4, 17, 19, 21, 52; feminism and, 4;
   hysteria and, 14–16, 18–19, 42;
   inductive tradition and, 44, 52–53,
   77, 135, 158, 169; self-analysis and,
   106; child abuse and, 124, 131–140,
   146
Seelig, B. J., 183, 184, 194, 197
Self-analysis legend: importance of, 2,

16, 19–20, 44, 49, 97–105, 106–117,
   171–173, 179–180; perilous journey
   in, 28–29, 101–104, 114–115; mystique of, 99–105, 106, 114–117; suffering in, 103, 115, 117; secrecy in,
   105–110, 112, 114; criticism of, 106,
   180; evidence and, 107–111, 116;
   expert observer in, 110–111, 114,
   116
SEPtrans, 188–189
Serial processing, 170
Severinus, 51
Sexual abuse: childhood, 3–4, 14–19,
   42, 124, 131–140, 146, 158; results
   of, 14–19, 42; universality of, 18–20.
   See also Seduction theory
Sexuality: infantile, 3–4, 10–11, 14–22,
   42, 102, 106, 124, 131–140, 146,
   158, 169; masculine, 22, 174–177;
   importance of, 150, 151; male hero
   and, 175–176; feminine, 176–177
Shadowing, 174
Signature analysis. *See Doctrine of Sig-*
   natures
Signs, 54–60. *See also Doctrine of Sig-*
   natures
Simile, 78, 127
Similitudes: signs and, 56–58; types of,
   58–63; clinical practice and, 61–68,
   156; importance of, 66–68, 138
Simon, Bennett, 22–23, 24, 81–82, 84
Singular solution, 121–122, 123, 138
Skinner, B. F., 85
Smith, Henry, 183, 184
Social class, 166–167
Social constructionism, 86
Sophocles, 10
Southern, R. W., 57
Specimen cases: impact of, 1–3, 30–31,
   34, 40–41, 48–49, 91–93, 97,
   110–111, 115–116, 145–147,
   155–158; credibility of, 36–38,
   52–54, 67–68, 72–74, 77, 91–93,
   103, 114, 116, 146–154, 179; core,
   39–41, 45–54, 56, 67–68, 71–74,
   88–94, 97, 110–116, 129–130,
   134–139, 145, 147, 150, 155–158,
   179; interchangeable, 48–49, 56,

113–114; atypical, 50, 124, 129, 135, 147, 152, 157–158; contingent features of, 53–54, 60, 67–68, 72–74, 90, 94, 120–121; necessary features of, 53–54, 66, 67–68, 91, 120; description of, 89–91, 120, 129–130, 134–135, 201

Speech patterns, 186–194, 197, 198

Spencer, J. H., Jr., 194

Standard Edition (Freud), 46–47, 79, 95–96, 109; as sacred text, 117, 151–152, 181; Preface, 181; new translation, 181–182

State, 57, 65

Steele, R. S., 107

Stein, Martin, 72–73, 80

Stoller, Robert, 90, 94

Stolorow, R. D., 170–171

Strachey, James, 2, 21, 93, 169, 181

Strether, Lambert, 131

Subliminal stimule, 188

Substance, 57

Sulloway, Frank, 44, 47, 101, 102–103, 106, 147, 163

Superego, 22

Syllepsis, 138

Symbiotic phase, 173–174

Symbols. *See* Signs

Sympathy, 59, 60, 63, 64

Target object. *See* Specimen cases

Tempkin, Owsei, 60

Thick description, 89, 120, 147. *See also Enargia*

Thurneisser, Leonhard, 126–127

Time, 57, 62

Toews, John E., 21, 42–44

Topographic surface, 183, 184

Training analysis, 163

Transference, 4, 61, 91, 106, 140, 156, 160, 188, 191, 196, 197

Transformation, 54–60, 62, 64, 137, 138, 154

Traumdeutung, Die (Freud), 16, 21, 25, 104, 113; metaphors in, 27–29, 31, 35–36, 78–79, 85, 97; as descriptive science, 29–31, 34–38, 42–48, 56, 97; pictorial language in, 31, 33–36, 97;

credibility of, 34–38, 46–48, 97–98, 108; specimen set in, 45, 46–48, 56; signature analysis and, 56; infantile wishes in, 98–99; self-analysis and, 101, 102, 109; first edition, 109; second edition, 109–110

Tribich, D., 118

Tropes, 78–79, 85, 86, 108–109, 130. *See also* Rhetoric; Rhetorical figures

Tropics of Discourse (White), 164

Truth, 39–41, 46, 105, 109, 125, 139; general laws and, 67–74, 91, 120, 126–127, 154; plausibility vs., 70; narrative, 78, 79–80, 90, 118–120, 129, 135, 158–159, 172–173, 178–179; historical, 79. *See also* Coherence theory; Correspondence theory

Tutankhamen, 167, 168

Twain, Mark, 25, 174–177

Unambiguous reference, 164–165

Uncompelled consensus, 3, 126, 139, 140, 194

Unconscious, 4, 17, 43, 95, 128, 150; relation to conscious, 21, 45, 160; self-analysis and, 28, 100–104, 106, 110–111; inaccessibility of, 62, 84, 86, 165–166; described, 84; metaphor and, 84, 86, 96, 165–166; underworld and, 104; timeless, 167, 168, 169; analytic surface and, 184

Uniformity of Nature, Principle of (Hume), 54

Universalism, 162–163

Unwitting interpretation, 11, 73

Valéry, Paul, 88–89

Validation, 11, 104, 113–114, 116, 128, 132, 158, 160, 165–166, 179–181, 195, 199

Van der Hoop, J. H., 151

Vanishing referent, 82, 129, 146, 164–166, 194–195

Vesalius, 51

Vickers, Brian, 34, 42, 50, 77–78, 125, 126–127

Viderman, Serge, 184

Walker, D. P., 127
Wallerstein, R. S., 82–83, 84, 198–199
Waugaman, R. M., 149–150, 153–156, 157, 158, 160, 162
We, the Tikopia (Firth), 31–32
Westfall, R. S., 41
White, Hayden, 164
'Wild' analysis, 71, 166
Williams, Miriam, 131–140, 146, 157, 158, 162
Windholz, Michael, 189
Winnicott, D. W., 156

Wisdom, 84–85, 200–204
Wish fulfillment, 2, 11, 20–21, 35, 45, 79, 98–100, 103, 110, 129
Wissen, 200
Wittgenstein, Ludwig, 195
Workable surface, 185, 193, 199
Wurmser, Leon, 82

Young male hero myth, 174–177, 178

Zweig, Stefan, 167